The Politics of Health Information

Bedford Way Papers

ISSN 0261—0078

The Politics of Health Information

Beating Heart Disease as a case study in the production of Health Education Council publications

Wendy Farrant and Jill Russell

Bedford Way Papers 28
Institute of Education, University of London
distributed by Turnaround Distribution Ltd

First published in 1986 by the Institute of Education, University of London,
20 Bedford Way, London WC1H 0AL.

Distributed by Turnaround Distribution Ltd., 27 Horsell Road,
London N5 1XL (telephone: 01-609 7836).

The opinions expressed in these papers are those of the authors and do not necessarily reflect those of the publisher.

ISBN   0   85473   260   8

British Library Cataloguing in Publication Data

Farrant, Wendy
  The politics of health information: Beating heart disease as a case study in the production of Health Education Council publications. — (Bedford Way papers, ISSN 0261-0078; 28)
  1. Health education — Government policy — Great Britain
  I. Title   II. Russell, Jill
  III. Health Education Council. Beating heart disease   IV. University of London,
  Institute of Education   V. Series
  613'.07'041   RA440.3.G7

  ISBN 0-85473-260-8

Printed in Great Britain by Reprographic Services
Institute of Education, University of London.
Typesetting by Joan Rose

151/152-001-076-1186

Contents

This report is based on research funded by the Health Education Council. The views expressed in the report are those of the authors, and do not necessarily represent the views of the Council.

Wendy Farrant is lecturer in Health Education in the Academic Department of Community Medicine at St Mary's Hospital Medical School, University of London. She was senior research officer of the Health Education Publications Project in the department of Health and Welfare Studies at the Institute of Education, University of London.

Jill Russell is research fellow in the Social Research Unit of University College, Cardiff. She was research officer of the Health Education Publications Project in the department of Health and Welfare Studies at the Institute of Education, University of London.

Foreword

As this Bedford Way Paper was about to be published, an event occurred which has given new force to the thesis which it advances, that government views are overriding in the determination of Health Education Council policies. On 21 November 1986 the Secretary of State for Social Services announced in Parliament that, from 1 April 1987, the Health Education Council is to be dissolved and will be reconstituted as a 'Special Health Authority as an integral part of the National Health Service'. The statement suggests that the new Authority 'will initially assume the current respnsibilities of the Health Education Council and will, from an early date, be given the major executive responsibility for public education about AIDS'.

An article in the *Guardian* of 22 November carried the headline 'Health Education Council scrapped' and quoted a 'senior HEC official' as saying that, 'It will almost certainly mean a diminution of direct political campaigning. The Health Authority clearly won't campaign against the Government.' The same article reports a Council member as observing that 'the emphasis will be on education rather than lobbying'.

The episode affords a dramatic illustration of what this Bedford Way Paper calls 'shifting boundaries' in the constraints under which the Health Education Council works. This latest shift must be of great concern to all those professionally involved in health education. The comments quoted in the *Guardian* echo one of the informants quoted in this volume who speaks of 'the political impossibility, at the current time, of the HEC being able to be intellectually more honest'. If this was so under current contraints (as the volume demonstrates), how much worse is it likely to be under the new arrangements?

Ironically, the front pages of national newspapers at the time of the announcement were dominated by thè testimony given in an Australian court by Sir Robert Armstrong, Secretary to the Cabinet, in the case in which the British Government is seeking to prevent publication of a book about MI5. A new catchphrase has come into popular use as a result of Sir Robert's admission that in an earlier cross-examination he had been 'economical with the truth'.

The phrase epitomizes a modern, sophisticated form of propaganda, in health education as elsewhere, in which there is, as this volume shows, 'selective presentation of scientific evidence to support an official position'. This study helps us to see in what directions 'being economical with the truth' is leading us in health promotion: a conspiracy of silence on deprivation as a factor in social inequalities in health; a conspicuous avoidance of education for social action and a favouring of education for individual change; and a concentration on health messsages that foreshorten and oversimplify complex and difficult issues.

I hope that publication of this Bedford Way Paper will alert wider audiences to the dilemmas and encourage the debates that are essential on these issues.

Alan Beattie
Director, Health Education Publications Project and
Head of Health & Welfare Studies,
University of London Institute of Education,
26 November 1986

Preface

The research on which this paper is based was conducted as part of a three-year action research project (the Health Education Publications Project), housed at the University of London Institute of Education and funded by the Health Education Council (HEC). The project was jointly initiated by the Institute and by the HEC, with the aim of illuminating and informing as to the publications part of the HEC's work and suggesting practical proposals for change. It represented a collaborative attempt by a funding body and an academic institution to develop a style of research that would be able both to maintain the closest possible links to facilitate changes in the operational side of publications at the HEC itself and, at the same time, take advantage of a position of academic freedom of inquiry to develop an independent critique.

A confidential draft version of this paper was submitted to the HEC, in the form of an interim report, at the end of the second year of the Project (1983). The interim report was subsequently discussed at seminars and workshops of the British Sociological Association Medical Sociology Group, Cambridge University Child Care and Development Group, the London School of Hygiene and Tropical Medicine Department of Community Health, Oxford University Department of Community Medicine and General Practice, the Politics of Health Group, Thoms Coram Research Unit, and various health education officer forums.

The report became the subject of much discussion and debate within the HEC. It also provoked considerable interest outside the Council. It was clear from the feedback that we received at seminars and from individuals who commented on the draft report, that although the case study had a very specific focus (the production of an HEC booklet on heart disease), it was seen as raising questions that were pertinent to the work of people involved in health education policy, practice and research in a wide variety of contexts. In addition, readers for the Institute of

Education Publications Committee highlighted the relevance and interest of the case study for a more general audience of teachers and educationalists and others with an interest in the politics of information and knowledge. It was in recognition of this wide interest that the Institute of Education decided to approach the Health Education Council for permission to produce a revised version of the report as a Bedford Way Paper.

Given the potential sensitivity of much of the material contained in the report, the decision to release it for publication was clearly not an easy one for the HEC. We are therefore grateful to the Council for eventually allowing us to share with others some of our privileged insights into the world of HEC publications production.

As an action research initiative, the Health Education Publications Project was committed to a research practice that moved beyond examining, charting and documenting, to exploring the possibilities for change. In the final report of the Project[1] we discuss a number of examples of good practice that reflect the increasing commitment of the HEC, over the course of the project, to challenge some of the problematic traditional assumptions of health education publications production that were highlighted by this case study. At the same time, we have documented the constraints which militate against such positive innovations being easily incorporated into long-term policy. We hope that by extending the debate outside the HEC, this paper will play a part in facilitating an understanding of the dilemmas and contradictions that confront individuals attempting to work within these constraints to produce health education publications aimed at shifting the pattern of distribution of information (and thereby, ultimately, challenging the balance of power and control) between different groups in our society.

The research would not have been possible without the co-operation and active encouragement of the HEC publications section — in particular Nancy Kohner, Adrian Pollitt and Rosie Leyden. Their close involvement with the aims and work of the project has enabled action research to develop as it in theory always should, but in practice rarely does.

The project Director, Alan Beattie, and the project steering committee have always provided pertinent advice and eased the often painful process of decision making by sharing it with us. Apart from the staff of the HEC publications division named above, other members of the steering committee at the time of the research discussed in this paper were: Linda Ewles, Hilary Graham, Karen Greenwood, John Harris and Jill Rakusen. Our thanks to all of them.

Nadia Quinlan, the project Administrative Secretary, was a constant source of help, support and humour.

Simon Smail and Simon James kindly helped to arrange access to the research samples for the pretesting of *Beating Heart Disease*. The research respondents gave us a mass of rich data in their views on heart disease and health education. We should like to thank all respondents for the time and effort they gave to being interviewed.

We should also like to thank the individual officers from the HEC and from the BBC, whom we interviewed and those who made information available for the production of this report.

We are grateful to Denis Baylis, Denis Lawton, John White, and, of course, Alan Beattie, for their part in the delicate negotiations with the HEC about publication of this paper.

Our thinking about coronary prevention has been stimulated by the many useful discussions that we have had with Mel Bartley, David St George, and the Women and Food subgroup of the Politics of Health Group (Jenny Harding, Anne Karpf, Ruth Parish, Linnie Price, Helena Sheiham, Julie Shephard, Gill Smith and Nancy Worcester). Many other people have contributed to this paper by sharing with us their thoughts and experiences, providing information, and commenting on drafts. In particular we should like to thank Lee Adams, Nick Black, Nick Dorn, Mary Ann Elston, Merrill Evans, Bill Mayblin, Alan Maryon Davis, Jim McKewan, Jerry Morris, Roslin Pill, Jane Randall, Hazel Slavin, Gill Shaw, Ian Sutherland, Keith Tones and Sheila White.

Our thanks also to Helen Edwards, Margaret Simpson and Marcella Taylor for their help with the typing of this paper.

We are grateful to the Health Education Council for their financial support of the research.

The views expressed in the report are, of course, those of the authors, and do not necessarily reflect the views of any other individual or institution.

W.F.   J.R.
July, 1986

Chapter 1
Introduction

Don't wait until its too late. Do something now. Take some advice and help yourself to a healthier heart . . . By smoking, eating too much of the wrong food and not getting enough exercise you could be gambling with the health of your heart . . . It's never too late to change. Stop smoking, eat sensibly and learn to relax. You'll not only feel fitter than you've felt for years. You'll be giving yourself and your heart a new lease of life.

Beating Heart Disease, Health Education Council, 1984.

This quotation is an extract from a free booklet for the general public on coronary heart disease (CHD) produced by the Health Education Council (HEC) — a government sponsored organization with national responsibility for health education in England, Wales and Northern Ireland. The quotation and the booklet itself reflect and encapsulate the now familiar themes of what has been termed 'the conventional, largely "do-it-yourself", approach to health education [which] suggests that if individuals wish to live longer and healthier the main priority is for them to alter their lifestyles'.[1]

The purpose of this paper is to use the production of the HEC booklet *Beating Heart Disease* as a case study in the politics of health information and health education. The observations that we shall be presenting are drawn from primary and secondary sources of data, collected as part of the work of the Health Education Publications Project (HEPP) — a policy-oriented action research project concerned with evaluating the processes of production, distribution and use of HEC leaflets, booklets and posters.[2]

The production of *Beating Heart Disease* provides a useful focus for a critical examination of government-sponsored health education policy and practice. In terms of its content and style of communication, and the social relations of its production, *Beating Heart Disease* epitomizes the conventional, individual-behaviour oriented approach to health education, as defined at the beginning of this chapter. Within current health education debate, this conventional approach has become the subject of increasing scrutiny and criticism. The nature of this criticism has been covered in detail elsewhere.[3] The limitations of conventional health education can be summarized as:

1. the 'victim blaming' individualistic orientation, which fails to take adequate account of the social and economic determinants of ill health and health-related behaviour that lie outside individual control;

2. the 'top down' approach to planning of health education interventions, and consequent lack of relevance of many health education activities to the health concerns, experiences, and self-defined health information needs of the 'target audience';

3. the prescriptive style of health education communication, which can be seen as reinforcing the traditional 'active-and-dominant expert, passive-and-dependent-client' model of interaction, that has been identified as a barrier to people acting individually and collectively to take control of their own health.

Alternative strategies have focused on the potential of health education as a vehicle for social as well as for individual change, and on its potential for individual and community empowerment. A study of the production of *Beating Heart Disease* provides an opportunity for charting some of the assumptions, value judgements and constraints that underlie the HEC's continued failure adequately to respond to this critique of conventional health education in their publications policy.

Furthermore, given the significance of HEC publications in reflecting and disseminating an official ideology of health, and given the nature of scientific evidence and knowledge in the field of CHD, the production of *Beating Heart Disease* is a pertinent case example for highlighting wider issues in the politics of health information and health knowledge. In a recent inaugural lecture,[4] Professor Michael Marmot noted how individual scientists' interpretation of the evidence on diet and CHD appears to derive 'as much from ideological or political belief as from scientific judgement'. He also cited examples from the history of CHD research to illustrate the phenomena whereby 'When facts collide with theories, scientists are far more likely to discard or explain away the facts than the theory', and, 'If facts are inconvenient, scientists may even prefer to change them rather than reject the original theory'. Marmot's observation that health information (like any other branch of scientific knowledge) is politically defined, and our illustration of his observation in this paper, is not, of course, in any way original. What we hope to contribute by this detailed case study of the production of *Beating Heart Disease* is an insight into the political processes at work.

Our approach to evaluation of the HEC publications enterprise has been cited by Beattie as an example of the evaluative strategies of both 'appraising institutional agendas' and, at the same time 'analysing client's perspectives'.[5] It is an approach that begins with a recognition of the power that education, knowledge and information carry with them, in the field of health and medicine as anywhere else. By focusing, at one and the same time, on those producing and providing information on health and on the intended recipients of that information, it enables an evaluation of health education publications to describe and make visible the distribution of information (and thereby, ultimately power and control) between those particular groups in our society. It is in this sense that we see this case study as having a broader relevance for a sociology of health information.

We begin this paper (Chapter 2) by outlining the scope of the scientific debate on the aetiology and prevention of CHD. In so doing, we aim to illustrate salient features in the social construction of knowledge. Before examining how the HEC used and made sense of the scientific evidence, we present a brief review of the process of initiation and production of *Beating Heart Disease,* in order to examine the question of who controls decisions about HEC publications (Chapter 3). We then move on to discuss some of the factors that lay behind the decision of the HEC to confine the contents of the booklet to practical advice for individuals, and the implications of this decision making for the translation of scientific evidence (Chapter 4). In Chapter 5 we present some observations from the small-scale pretesting we conducted on part of the booklet, that suggest a lay perspective on disease aetiology and prevention very different from that presented by the HEC. We explore the implications of this difference in perspective for respondents' evaluation of *Beating Heart Disease*. Finally (in Chapter 6) we relate the themes emerging from this case study to wider issues in coronary prevention and health education.

Chapter 2
Coronary Heart Disease and the Scientific Evidence: the Scope of the Debate

It is clear that whilst we do not fully understand the causes of CHD we do know how to reduce considerably the risk of developing it. (DHSS, 1981)[1]

Despite the considerable uncertainty that surrounds many aspects of CHD, there is no shortage of enthusiastic proposals for action. (Open University Health and Disease Course, 1985)[2]

Much as we might like to think otherwise, it is not yet possible to prevent CHD in the community, let alone in an individual. (Oliver, 1982)[3]

In spite of enormous investments of time, money and manpower, there is still no consensus on the optimum strategy for preventing heart disease. (*The Times Health Supplement,* 1982)[4]

The production of health education material generally involves the translating of knowledge into information that can be communicated to a lay audience and presented in the form of practical advice. However, as the above quotes indicate, scientific knowledge about the aetiology and prevention of CHD is by no means unequivocal, immediately rendering translation of that knowledge into preventive advice problematic. Before describing the production of *Beating Heart Disease*, we shall briefly outline, in this chapter, the scope of evidence available to the HEC about CHD aetiology and prevention. In so doing, we shall illustrate salient features of the social construction of scientific and medical knowledge.[5] We shall suggest that the problematic nature of knowledge on CHD aetiology and prevention can, in part at least, be attributed to the difficulties, and some would say inappropriateness, of fitting what is currently known about CHD into a conventional medical model of disease aetiology and intervention. We shall go on to examine the challenging, and potentially threatening, nature of some of the scientific evidence for medical and other vested interests.

We should stress that our aim in this section is to outline the breadth and complexities of debate, rather than to provide a comprehensive review of the current state of evidence. In so doing, we shall inevitably highlight areas where dissension and confusion, real or manipulated, exist. This is not to deny the significance of consensus and common ground on many of the general principles of the CHD debate.

Personal risk factors
The leading predictors of CHD are conventionally recognized as cigarette smoking, an elevated blood cholesterol level and raised blood pressure.[6] Other factors that are widely considered to be directly or indirectly associated with CHD include obesity and physical inactivity. Major national and international reports[7] suggest that a consensus of expert opinion regarding the causal significance of these classic risk factors has now been reached. It is argued that 'the stage is now set for vigorous application of existing knowledge to reduce CHD incidence and mortality'.[8] Preventive strategies have been implemented aimed at reducing the classic risk factors through such measures as smoking control, promotion of healthy nutrition and exercise and screening and treatment for high blood pressure.

Even though there is substantial agreement among experts about the importance of the classic risk factors in the aetiology and the prevention of CHD, there are still, as Marmot points out, 'numerous pieces of the puzzle which do not fit neatly into place'.[9] For example, associations (e.g. between dietary fats, blood cholesterol and CHD mortality) derived from international comparisons of data *between* countries do not always hold *within* countries.[10] There also exists international epidemiological data where associations between the classic risk factors and incidence of CHD do not hold — where a decline in CHD mortality is taking place despite an increase in certain risk factors[11] and conversely, where the incidence of CHD is increasing despite risk factor reduction.[12] Furthermore, whilst the 'conventional' risk factors for CHD have been shown to account for part of the difference in incidence of CHD between different populations, they also leave a great deal of the variance of the disease unexplained:

. . . prospective epidemiological studies often show that coronary risk factors can account for only 50-60 per cent of the total variance of the disease within the period of observation. Indeed in one such study, on the relationship between employment grade, coronary risk factors and CHD in British civil servants, only 40 per cent of the difference in CHD between employment grades could be accounted for by risk factors that were measured on entry to the study.[13]

In addition, as noted in the recent report on *Diet and Cardiovascular Disease* by the DHSS Committee on Medical Aspects of Food Policy:[14]

Multiple risk factor intervention trials have not shown convincing evidence of benefit.

These trials have attempted to show, without any clear success, that modification of the classic risk factors leads to a significant reduction in CHD mortality. As an article in *Medical News*[15] concluded:

. . . though the results [of the Oslo trial, the Multiple Risk Factor Intervention Trial (MRFIT) and the WHO European Collaborative Trial] are not incompatible with the theory that risk factor intervention modifies the incidence of CHD, they can scarcely be said to be compatible with it either.

The disappointing results of the multiple risk intervention trials does not, of course, deny the useful information for epidemiologists and health educationalists produced by these trials, nor, as the above quote suggests, does it necessarily negate the hypothesis tested by the trials. Rather, such results indicate the need for caution and a broader perspective than hitherto adopted by the majority involved in the CHD prevention debate:

There is a widespread view that epidemiologic studies have made such a significant contribution to the elucidation of factors that put an individual at risk of developing CHD that it is time to take action in preventing the disease. Laudably, the action in the United States and Europe is initially taking the form of trials aimed at testing the effects of cessation of smoking and reducing blood pressure and serum lipid levels on subsequent morbidity and mortality. However, the commitment to these large-scale, complex, multi-center intervention trials has assumed massive proportions, to the comparative exclusion of further research into the aetiology of CHD. . . It is important that current ideas be put to the test as the intervention trials are doing, but it is also important that further research be conducted into this area if major inroads are to be made into the social and medical problem of coronary heart disease.[16]

General susceptibility

The distribution of deaths from CHD, as with virtually every other cause of mortality in our society, is strongly and inversely related to social class.[17] The findings of the Whitehall Study (a major longitudinal study of CHD mortality in male civil servants) suggest that a large part of this social class difference in CHD mortality remains unexplained by the conventional risk factors.[18] Furthermore, even in so far as differences in CHD mortality between social groups *can* be attributed to differences in personal risk factors, it still remains necessary to explore *why* the difference in risk factors between social groups exists. As the authors of a recent article on the Whitehall Study noted:

> It is not sufficient to conclude that these risk factors provide part of the explanation of social differences in mortality. Attention should be concentrated on the reasons for social class differences in smoking, in obesity, in leisure-time physical activity, and on what can be done about them. This is an urgent task of public health.[19]

Gender differences in CHD mortality similarly parallel more general differences in mortality between the sexes, with higher mortality rates for men than for women. Elevated CHD mortality rates have also been recorded for certain ethnic minority groups — for example, UK Asians. Whilst CHD research has primarily focused on white males, the evidence that is available suggests that gender and ethnic differences in CHD mortality cannot adequately be explained by conventional risk factors.[20]

As evidence of the limited explanatory power of the conventional risk factors accumulates, researchers are beginning to look further afield — and particularly towards the wider psychosocial and socioeconomic environment — to explain the variance in incidence of CHD. The list of factors associated with CHD continues to grow:

> One review listed twenty-two such items as 'some of the factors' that have been statistically associated with the frequency of the disease, and there are no doubt others waiting discovery.[21]

Some researchers are fundamentally questioning the primacy of conventionally accepted personal risk factors, and are utilizing the concept of general susceptibility to explain not only the difference in CHD mortality between different social groups, but also the similarity in social distribution of CHD and of other diseases. Within this framework, a model of CHD aetiology has been hypothesized that locates the primary cause of CHD (and therefore the appropriate point for intervention) in the wider social and economic environment, and utilizes the concept of chronic psychosocial stress as the major linking factor between an individual's environment and his or her cardiovascular system.[22] The hypothesis of chronic social stress as a primary factor in the aetiology of CHD provides a framework for interpreting not only the significance of conventional CHD risk factors,[23] but also, the social distribution of CHD and CHD-related behaviour (discussed above), and the relationship of CHD to such variables as unemployment,[24] fluctuations in the business cycle,[25] work pressure and occupational organization,[26] and the 'Type A' personality pattern, characterized by hard-driving competitiveness, unrelieved work pressure and inability to relax.[27]

Vested interests
It should be clear from the above discussion that there remain real areas of contention and dissension in the current debate on CHD. The picture of confusion has certainly been exacerbated, however, by those with vested interests in the direction of the CHD debate.

A central area of debate within the medical literature on CHD prevention has concerned the appropriateness of 'high risk' versus 'population' strategies for risk factor reduction. A high-risk strategy attempts to identify and bring preventive care to individuals within a population who are at special risk of CHD, whereas a population strategy focuses on the *whole population* as the target for intervention. The WHO Expert Committee on Prevention of Coronary Heart Disease,[28] whilst accepting the need for a high-risk strategy, argued strongly for the importance of this being complemented by a population strategy aimed at

> altering the lifestyle and environmental characteristics, and their social and economic determinants, that are the underlying causes of mass CHD.

The rationale for the WHO Expert Committee's concept of a population strategy has been explained in detail by Geoffrey Rose[29] (Chairman of the Expert Committee). Rose has illustrated how the limiting of intervention to high-risk individuals would make insufficient impact on population rates of CHD, given that most cases of CHD come from the large group of the population at 'moderate' risk. Furthermore, epidemiological evidence has shown that the precision of prediction of individuals at high risk from the classic risk factors is not great.[30] Such limitations of a high-risk approach have led many to the conclusion that a mass strategy is inherently the only answer to a mass disease.[31]

The importance of intervening at the level of the underlying 'social and economic determinants' of mass CHD has been explained by Rose[32] partly in terms of:

> . . . what we might call the prevention paradox — *'a measure that brings large benefits to the community offers little to each participating individual'.* It implies that we should not expect too much from individual health education. People will not be motivated to any great extent to take our advice, because there is little in it for each of them . . . to influence mass behaviour we must look to its mass determinants which are largely economic and social.

The WHO Expert Committee on Community Prevention and Control of Cardiovascular Diseases[33] emphasizes that strategies for prevention

> must be broad based and must involve a wide range of community interests and policy makers; the medical aspects of prevention are considered within a broad political and social framework.

The broad-based strategy of prevention advocated by the WHO Expert Committee includes, for example, controls over the food, agricultural and tobacco industries. However, the Committee also notes that such measures are likely to be 'resisted by vested interests' and emphasizes that

> government, administrators and policy makers must facilitate and promote favourable conditions for prevention, whilst restraining those vested interests that obstruct prevention.

The role of vested interests in attempting to influence the direction of the CHD debate within the UK, was addressed in the TV series *Plague of Hearts* (for which *Beating Heart Disease* was produced as back-up material). O'Donnell, the presenter of the series, argued that:

> International opinion is now agreed on the risk factors for CHD, but we [Britain] have no agreed national policy for dealing with them. We still have powerful lobbies, the tobacco industry, the dairy industry, who deny the existence of the evidence.

Government departments, too, can be seen to represent economic interests. This was clearly illustrated by the Department of Health and Social Security's (DHSS) reaction to the report of the National Advisory Committee on

Nutrition Education (NACNE) produced around the time of our research on *Beating Heart Disease*.[34] To quote from the *Lancet:*

> . . . the [food] industry apparently disliked much of what it read [in the NACNE report] and seems to have got the Department [DHSS] to suppress or at any rate delay the report.[35]

Furthermore, the 'population' versus 'high risk' preventive strategy debate, within the medical literature, has, in part, to be seen in the context of the medical profession's own interests in keeping coronary prevention within medical control and within a conventional paradigm of medical intervention. One of the arguments that has been advanced in favour of a high-risk strategy of CHD prevention is that it offers for physicians (and patients) a more familiar and comfortable model of disease and medical practice. The WHO Expert Committee note that 'Doctors often lack the training and hence also the motivation to enlarge their responsibilities beyond the care of the sick.'[36] However, Rose points out that much harder to overcome than this general lack of physician motivation for preventive health care, 'is the enormous difficulty for medical personnel to see health as a population issue and not merely as a problem for individuals'.[37] Thus, whilst epidemiological theory points towards a population approach to CHD prevention, reviews of current practice and initiatives in the medical literature on CHD prevention suggest an emphasis by the medical profession on the role of high-risk screening strategies within a medical setting.

A far greater challenge to conventional medical thought is provided by the general susceptibility model of CHD aetiology referred to above. The hypothesis of chronic social stress as a primary factor in disease aetiology is not a new phenomenon.[38] It has never, however, been credited with orthodox attention. Selye, writing about this hypothesis in the 1950s, observed 'aversion is an integral part of the story of stress, because . . . stress is an abstraction'.[39] Marmot recently summed up the aversion of the medical profession to stress research as follows:

> We cannot define stress, we cannot measure it (stress to one person is stimulus to another) and hence by implication, stress does not exist. If the scientists cannot define or measure it, it can be ruled out of discussions on prevention.[40]

Marmot's own research on stress and CHD has challenged the notion that stress cannot be defined or measured and he has argued forcibly for the role of stress in CHD to be given the attention he believes it deserves:

> Stress needs to be brought into the scientific discourse on prevention of coronary disease. Attempts can be made to define it, to measure it, to study it. It can be studied scientifically, one can attempt to moderate its effects and evaluate those attempts. It is a serious discussion that should take place in a scientific and public health context.[41]

However, the 'aversion' to the concept of chronic social stress as a primary factor in disease aetiology can be seen as extending beyond such methodological considerations. It has been argued that integrating the concept of social stress into an aetiological model of CHD, would ultimately require a major reformulation of the theoretical as well as the methodological perspectives that guide medical research in this area. It would suggest the need to focus research more on *relationships between people,* and between individuals and the social environment, rather than the effect commodities such as smoking or diet have on individuals. Furthermore, this alternative model of CHD aetiology ultimately challenges orthodox medical practice by locating the appropriate point for intervention within the social and economic environment:

> . . . a primary prevention programme [based on such a model] would likely focus on the modification of the psychosocial environment which has induced the [body's] metabolic imbalance . . .[42]

Eyer [43] presents data on hypertension as a disease of modern society that (he suggests)

> . . . imply that major social changes are necessary to prevent modern hypertension . . . there would certainly [need to] be major redefinitions of the nature of production and productivity, and major reorganization of lifetime work patterns.

It has been suggested[44] that the reasons for the slowness of the medical profession to recognize stress in the aetiology of CHD lie both in the challenge of such a model of disease, and also in a feeling that its recognition would take CHD prevention firmly outside medicine and into the socio-economic system.

Current approaches to CHD prevention within the UK[45] would appear to make little concession to the need to address the underlying social and economic determinants of *inequalities* in CHD between social groups. The emphasis (both within 'high risk' and 'population' strategies) is primarily upon changing individual lifestyles. Within this focus, local food and smoking policies have made some progress towards effecting changes in the wider environment. However, the measures emphasized (e.g. increasing the nutritional value of institutional food, introduction of 'no-smoking' areas, etc.) generally bypass the underlying determinants of *inequalities* in nutrition and smoking behaviour (i.e. poverty, stress associated with adverse living and working conditions, and so on).[46]

In so far as the underlying social and economic determinants of inequalities in CHD *have* been accepted as aetiologically significant, they are often dismissed as irrelevant to or a diversion from prevention. Thus Le Fanu — an active medical journalist in the CHD debate — draws attention to the significance of the relationship between social class and CHD but dismisses this as an inappropriate focus for health education and, in any case, 'essentially unalterable'. Furthermore, the 1982 WHO Expert Committee[47] acknowledges that:

> Other characteristics of social organization and personal status have been thought to aggravate CHD, though none is considered a primary determinant. It is possible that some of these factors might be favourably modified with respect to occupation, living conditions, working hours, education and socioeconomic status.

However, in the Committee's recommendations for prevention, no reference was made to these factors, which can be regarded as major determinants of chronic social stress. On the contrary:

> The Expert Committee noted the danger that public and professional misconceptions about 'stress', whereby it is assigned a primary role in the genesis of CHD, may divert attention from demonstrated needs in prevention.

This view was essentially reiterated in the 1986 report of the WHO Expert Committee on Community Prevention and Control of Cardiovascular Diseases:[48]

> Stress related to social and occupational factors is thought to be associated with an increased risk of cardiovascular diseases. This subject is potentially important, but a causal relationship and the possibility of effective intervention have not been demonstrated. Therefore, at the present time, no recommendations can be made regarding the possibility of reducing the risk of cardiovascular diseases by acting on stress factors.

The boundaries of the CHD debate are thus set in such a way as to leave unchallenged the social divisions which underly the unequal distribution of CHD within our society.

Chapter 3
Beating Heart Disease —
why and how it was produced

For the vast majority of users of HEC publications, professionals and 'consumers' alike, the preparation of any publication is largely a hidden and unknown process. However, if our task of evaluating HEC publications was to be comprehensive, it was essential carefully to monitor and record the process of initiation and production of publications, in order to gain an understanding of the institutional and organizational constraints within which publications are produced, and to explore the ways in which production decisions influence their content and style. A detailed analysis of the HEC publications production process is contained in the final report of the Health Education Publications project.[1] For present purposes we shall simply present a brief overview of the process of initiation and production of *Beating Heart Disease*. In so doing, we shall draw attention to those features of the production process that contributed to a 'top-down' style of working, whereby decisons about the initiation, content and style of the publication were taken 'from above', with no opportunity for any meaningful input from the target audience. In particular, we shall illustrate the professional, and specifically medical, control over decision making.

Our research on the production of *Beating Heart Disease* involved: interviews with staff of the HEC and BBC who were responsible for the initiation and production of the booklet; observation of consultations between the HEC Publications Division[2] and Medical Division;[3] monitoring of communications between the HEC and external consultants who were asked to comment on the booklet; observation of consultations between the HEC and graphic designers, plus interviews with the designers; monitoring of the proceedings of the HEC Coronary Heart Disease Programme Group, and monitoring of HEC Management Team and Council meetings at which the coronary heart disease booklet and Programme were discussed. Later in this chapter we shall explain how we also became involved in the 'pretesting' of the booklet on the target audience.

Throughout this and the following chapter we draw upon research data
we collected in these various ways, although issues of confidentiality make
it inappropriate in most cases for quotes to be attributed.

Origination of the decision to produce *Beating Heart Disease*
The immediate impetus for the production of *Beating Heart Disease* was
a request from the BBC for back-up material to support a series of radio[4]
and BBC2 TV[5] programmes on CHD. This way of working (producing
support print for the BBC) represents a trend that began in the mid-1970s
and one that the HEC has, over the past few years, been increasingly committed to. As explained in the HEC Annual Report of 1981-1982[6]

> Television and print, used in combination with each other and with well
> organized back-up activity at local level offer what is potentially a highly
> effective means of health education.

The advantages of such collaboration from the viewpoint of the BBC were
explained to us as follows:

> . . . we are getting free support literature, and that's very important for
> us . . . and they [the HEC] are getting a national focus of an educational
> nature.

However, the acceptance by the HEC of the BBC's invitation of collaboration can, and must, also be located within broader policy at that
time — both inside and outside the HEC. Since 1982[7] the strategies,
objectives and planned activities in the HEC's main areas of work have
been co-ordinated and labelled as 'Programmes'. Although BBC production schedules meant that *Beating Heart Disease* was produced before the
HEC's Programme on the Prevention of CHD[8] had been finalized,
discussion and drafting of the Programme was well under way. In this
sense CHD was already identified as a key area of HEC initiative. The
significance of central government in shaping HEC priorities (in general,
and programme topics in particular) has been discussed elsewhere by
ourselves[9] and others.[10] In the case of the CHD Programme, there was
evidence of external pressure from the DHSS following their publication
of *Avoiding Heart Attacks*[11] for the HEC to intensify their CHD prevention activity. At the same time, the HEC CHD Programme can, to a large
extent, be seen as an extension of the HEC's 'Look After Yourself!' (LAY)
campaign of the late 1970s. Initiation of the CHD prevention programme

coincided with a felt need within the HEC 'to discover yet another way of highlighting and "lifting" the LAY campaign during another year'. It was suggested that the HEC was at a point when quite radical changes were required in LAY if it was not to become:

> a superficial irrelevance, 'a good idea at the time', or frankly, a bore . . . It will not be sufficient to continue to promote the basic messages (eat less and better, exercise more, stop smoking) without giving them a more pointed context. The campaign lacks 'a common enemy' to which people can relate and it would be helpful if a medical consensus were arrived at to allow HEC to link its messages more closely to CHD . . .

Development of the text

Beating Heart Disease was written by the HEC Publications Division from a medical brief prepared by the HEC Medical Division.

As is routine practice for the production of HEC publications, the text was developed in consultation with a range of 'experts' in the subject area. The consultants used for *Beating Heart Disease* consisted of three professors of community medicine or epidemiology, one professor of cardiology, a senior lecturer in general practice, a community physician, two representatives of the Coronary Prevention Group, and a representative of a clinical nutrition centre. Two of the consultants were also HEC Council members. In terms of the almost exclusive dependence on medical expertise (as opposed to other disciplines), and in terms of their professional standing, the medical consultants used for *Beating Heart Disease* represented a fairly typical HEC list — somewhat longer than usual, perhaps because of the controversial nature of CHD prevention. As to how this list was drawn up, it was described to us as:

> . . . a question of pulling together the names of key people that one has worked with before or have been involved with from other organizations like the Coronary Prevention Group, or NACNE [National Advisory Committee on Nutrition Education], or been involved with at the various conferences or one simply has read that they are just key people in the field and read their papers. It was simply a question of consulting a rather select group to try and get as broad an opinion as possible without consulting so widely that the whole thing was completely bogged down.

For the HEC, it is this issue that ultimately lies behind the problematic nature of medical consultation — what to do with and how to make sense of a wide spectrum of medical opinion. The temptation, under such circumstances, is to canvass opinion in such a way as to get as much consensus as possible and to attempt to steer clear of issues where consensus cannot be reached. In the case of *Beating Heart Disease* the problems of consultation were further exacerbated by tight time constraints,[12] by the controversial nature of CHD, and by the fact (mentioned earlier) that the booklet preceded publication of the CHD Programme.[13]

The other main group with whom consultation took place were health education officers (HEOs), represented through the HEC Health Education Officers' Publications Panel. Although it is often assumed that health education officers provide the link between the HEC and the consumer, our research[14] on HEOs has indicated that the majority of HEOs have very little direct contact with consumers, but rather see their role mainly as being to work with professionals. The role of the HEO Publications Panel was defined as 'facilitating field comment' on HEC publications, and as representing both health education officers and 'the relevant professionals in their area'.[15] The field comment included, in this instance (in addition to the Panel's own views and those of HEC colleagues), comments from a doctor, a district dietician, an ambulance officer, and a cardiologist.

As is more often than not the case with HEC publications, the views of the target audience — the general public — were not canvassed at all during the drafting of the text. This was represented to us as a major defect in the production process by those concerned:

> The constraints really were in the consultation process. We didn't consult as extensively as perhaps we should have done, we didn't consult as much as we needed to . . . all along we have made judgements about the target audience and which is best for the target audience. We haven't consulted any of the target audience . . . so it's a prime example of an HEC publication based on expert opinion, I suppose.

Development of the design

> Ideally draft copy writing would happen in conjunction with design, but we run into all sorts of problems with experts [consultants] at the draft copy stage and it's good to get them over before the design stage.

For reasons quoted above, design work does not usually begin on HEC publications until after the final text has been approved by the Medical

Division. In the case of *Beating Heart Disease* the designers first became involved after a draft of the text had been written. By then, the format, style and mood of the publication was already largely set:

> Full colour, highly illustrated, illustrations in the form of case history photographs, charts and diagrams, motivational and authoritative with a 'factual emphasis', 'straightforward . . . direct . . . serious without being alarming' in mood.

A central design feature was to be case histories in the form of 'reporting-style' commentaries. The designers and the HEC, however, had rather different views on the role and emphasis of such case histories. The designers envisaged that the photographs and quotes would cover a wide range of different sorts of people in a variety of real-life situations, for instance, a photo of dustmen smoking as an example of 'something actually showing people at risk in the sort of situations that create the risk'. However, the use of quotes was constrained by the HEC's belief that it was:

> . . . very important that the quotes clearly express what the text is trying to express, and we must get it right. The person has got to say the right thing otherwise it won't work.

Also, shortage of time meant that the HEC were forced to rely on personal contacts for case histories, leading to a predominance of white, middle-class people being represented in *Beating Heart Disease*. As a result of these factors, the final publication failed to live up to the expectations of the designers:

> We did rather hang everything on those photos . . . we realized we needed something to hang the booklet around visually, because charts and diagrams are not enough . . . It could have worked well but the photos didn't match up to the variety of people and situations that we'd originally envisaged and the quotes didn't do what we wanted . . . The photos were all of rather neat and tidy well-dressed people on their best behaviour . . . The quotes were used to underline points in the text. In the end they had a manipulative feel about them which people picked up . . . That was something we'd never envisaged. The idea for the quotes was that they would be a fascinating digression from text rather than being a slave to it . . . What they came out like was rather false-sounding, even though they were genuine quotes.

Another constraint that the designers were conscious of was the absence of any feedback from developmental research:

The other thing that we felt it suffered from was not having a clear idea of who we were designing for . . . There was no time to get together groups who represented the target audience, and the target audience — the general public — was so diverse anyway, so we ended up relying on graphic cliches . . . It came completely out of our heads, as graphic designers, and nothing was fed into that . . . no information could be gleaned [about views of the target audience] even from professionals . . . So it inevitably looks shallow and sterile . . . it lacks that element of developmental research.

Pretesting

Pretesting is a term taken from commercial marketing research. Within commercial marketing, pretesting theoretically refers to the final ('fine tuning') stage of a systematic programme of developmental consumer research:

. . . pretesting is the stage for final fine tuning of the material. It is *not* the stage for discovering errors in strategy, since by then expensive commitments will have been made to its production. The only way of ensuring this is for pretesting to follow problem definition and creative development research; where it is applied on its own, it runs the serious risk — and this is what happens most often in practice — of reporting gross errors in strategy or concept approach. It follows from this that dipping in and out of pretesting research, and applying it unsystematically only as a response to some external pressure is a waste of resources unless one is prepared to redevelop material from scratch.[16]

Within the HEC, however, 'prestesting' of publications is usually the first and only time that reactions of a target audience are canvassed, and takes place at a stage in the production process when it is too late for the publication to be significantly altered.

Pretesting of *Beating Heart Disease* was scheduled to take place alongside design development. By this stage the text had already been finalized and approved by the HEC Medical Division. So, even assuming a commitment to take account of the reactions of the target audience, it would have been extremely difficult for the content to be changed at this stage. In addition, as we have already discussed, time pressures on the production of design work precluded the possibility of design being meaningfully informed by developmental research. Despite these limitations, the HEC Committee that approved the proposal for the production of the booklet 'stressed the need for thorough pretesting before distribution because of the controversial nature of the issue'. Given that there was never any illusion that there would be time for pretesting to influence anything other than minor details of the design of the publication, this statement can only be understood in terms of the political advantages for the HEC of being able to *say* that pretesting has been done:

> . . . it's just reassurance more than anything, and afterwards it always helps, if we get criticized for something being inappropriate or unappealing . . . to be able to say that it was pretested and the results of that appear to be OK.[17]

It had been planned to commission a commercial market research agency to carry out the prestesting of *Beating Heart Disease*. Our offer to undertake this pre-testing research, as part of our broader research, was based on our recognition of the possibilities that it afforded for exploring further a number of issues central to the wider aims of the Health Education Publications Project. At the same time, we were able to produce some minor, but useful, pretesting findings that were fed back to the HEC and incorporated into the design of the final version of *Beating Heart Disease*.

As we shall discuss in Chapter 5, pretesting of *Beating Heart Disease* provided rich data on the depth and complexity of lay knowledge, beliefs and values regarding CHD aetiology and prevention; on the extent of match and mismatch between this lay perspective and the assumptions underlying the production of health education publications; and on the implications of the HEC's failure to take account of this lay perspective for respondents' evaluation of the health education message. In this sense, pretesting revealed fundamental problems concerning the style, content and underlying ideology of *Beating Heart Disease*.

Chapter 4
From Scientific Evidence to Booklet: the Health Education Council's translation of information

In Chapter 3 we documented the 'top-down' approach to the production of *Beating Heart Disease*, whereby decisions about the booklet's content and style of communication were taken by the HEC in consultation with professional advisors, with no meaningful input from representatives of the intended readership. In this chapter we shall look at the nature of the decision that were taken by the HEC, at some of the factors influencing such decisions, and at the problematic implications of this decision making for the presentation of information in *Beating Heart Disease*. Specifically, we shall look first at the HEC decision to focus information on practical advice to individuals and at some of the assumptions underlying such a decision — namely, the assumptions that: (1) it is not the role of HEC publications to educate for social change; (2) health education publications should reflect a consensus of medical opinion; (3) health education publications should be short and simple or they will not be read; and (4) the HEC must 'sell health'. We shall then look at the problems encountered by the HEC in attempting to translate population data relating to CHD aetiology and prevention into practical advice for individuals. Finally, we shall focus on the booklet's presentation of information on dietary goals and on stress in order to highlight the political constraints imposed by the HEC's structural position as a DHSS-funded quango, and to illustrate the ways in which information is steered towards a message that is both medically and politically acceptable.

The decision to focus information on practical advice to individuals
The overall aim of *Beating Heart Disease*, as defined in the HEC's formal proposal for the booklet, was 'to give information about the causes

and prevention of CHD'. However, as suggested in Chapter 2, the giving of such information cannot be assumed to be unproblematic. Rakusen[1] argues:

> ... the concept of 'complete' information is not only difficult to envisage, it is also ... potentially dangerous, fostering in us a false sense of what scientific and medical knowledge is really about.

In translating current knowledge about the aetiology and prevention of CHD into a health education message, the HEC was faced with a number of choices that have a bearing on more general aspects of health education policy. Central to this decision making were potential choices about the extent to which the booklet would address: (1) the evidence regarding the importance of social and economic factors in the causation and prevention of CHD; and (2) the areas of inconclusiveness, uncertainty and contention that exist within the scientific literature on CHD, and (related to this) the difficulties of translating the epidemiological evidence into practical advice for individuals.

As mentioned in Chapter 1, recent developments in health education theory have focused on the potential of health education as a vehicle for social, as well as for individual change. There has also been a shift towards more participatory and empowering strategies of health education. Within this changing concept of health education, we would suggest that the production of an HEC booklet on CHD potentially provided a valuable opportunity for offering readers information and skills to evaluate current knowledge relating to the aetiology and prevention of a major cause of mortality in our society, and to appraise the implications for individual and/or collective action.

It was clear from internal discussion documents that the role of socioeconomic factors in the aetiology and prevention of CHD was not unrecognized by the HEC. It was also apparent, as we shall discuss later in this chapter, that the HEC were well aware of the complexities of the scientific evidence relating to CHD prevention, and the difficulties of attempting to translate this evidence into useful advice for individuals. It was nevertheless explicit from the outset that the major objective of the booklet would be to give practical advice on how individuals could reduce their own risk of heart disease. So, even at the proposal stage of the publication, there was a selective definition of what information the booklet would contain — namely,

> advice on how to 'help yourself' to a healthier heart. (*Beating Heart Disease*, p.3.)

The lack of a social perspective in *Beating Heart Disease* is illustrated by the notable absence of any reference to the social class distribution of CHD. The short section of the booklet entitled 'Who gets heart disease?' is confined to information on international and regional comparisons of death rates from CHD. One professional consultant who commented on the draft text noted that this section reads:

> as though it is the geographical conditions that cause the higher rate rather than such things as the social class structure, higher unemployment and more stressful types of work.

A similar point, with reference to the final published version of *Beating Heart Disease*, was made in the following comment by a health education officer (in response to a HEPP questionnaire):

> [HEC publications] completely ignore any social/economic context within which health decisions are made and the major health influences which individuals have little/no control over. [They] completely ignore overwhelming evidence of class distribution of health (e.g. Black Report), e.g. recent very lavish *Beating Heart Disease* has virtually nothing on class distribution *within* UK. Deliberate concentration on *international* comparisons. As far as HEC publications go there is a conspiracy of silence on class inequalities in health.

The major section of the booklet entitled 'What causes heart disease' focuses on the personal risk factors of smoking, diet and high blood pressure. Within this focus, the responsibility for reducing risk factors is placed firmly upon the individual. There is no mention of, for example, the role of the food industry and tobacco industry in maintaining unhealthy consumption patterns, or of the social and economic factors (poverty, stress associated with adverse living and working conditions, and so on) that are related to social inequalities in diet, smoking, etc., and that militate against attempts at individual risk factor reduction. Exhortations to stop smoking, eat less fat, take more exercise, etc., are punctuated by assertions that 'experts believe' these measures to be effective for reducing the risk of CHD. Evaluation of the evidence is thus taken out of the reader's hands.

This decision to focus information on practical advice to individuals was related to assumptions about the role of HEC publications and about the information needs of the target audience.

1. *The assumption that it is not the role of HEC publications to challenge social policy*

At one level, the need for information for individuals to be supplemented by action directed at the social and economic determinants of mass CHD was not denied by the HEC. The final draft of the HEC Programme of Education for the Prevention of CHD,[2] for example, included the statement:

> The Council will seek to influence Government policy where it bears on health education with regard to CHD.

An earlier draft of the CHD programme had adopted the WHO Expert Committee[3] definition of a population strategy as one which is:

> . . . aimed at the general public, individually and collectively, decision makers and opinion formers, [to] encourage changes in the lifestyle *and environmental characteristics, and their social and economic determinants,* that are the underlying causes of mass CHD. (our italic)

However, by the final draft of the Programme the words 'and their social and economic determinants' had been omitted from this statement after advice from one consultant that the phrase was 'sufficiently implicit already'.

The TV series ('Plague of hearts') to which *Beating Heart Disease* was back-up material explicitly set out to:

> . . . examine the likely cause of the disease and see what changes individuals *or the government* could make to reduce its incidence.[4] (our italic)

The TV series included, for example, an analysis of the relationship between high national consumption of saturated fats and the profit motive of the dairy industry. However, matters of social policy were not considered to be appropriate subject matter for a health education booklet on CHD prevention aimed at the general public. To quote one HEC officer:

> . . . possibly [TV] programmes may be more designed to stimulate social policy change rather than booklets like the ones [the HEC] produce which I think are primarily, individually-oriented and are used that way by the people . . . These booklets are not designed to influence the politicians — that is a different thing. . . . if you want to tackle food policies you do it

in a different way, not through individuals who are concerned about heart disease . . . [and] if you are going to tackle social class inequalities in health you are not going to tackle it by a booklet on heart disease, or indeed a booklet on any other disease.

It was not, in fact, unknown at the time of our research on *Beating Heart Disease* for the HEC to argue for social change in their free publications aimed at the general public. The HEC leaflet on fluoridation of water supplies, entitled 'Is this what you want for your child?', ends with the statement:

Make your support of water fluoridation known. Write to: Your local Councillor/Your Member of Parliament/The Chairman of your Area Health Authority/The Secretary of your Community Health Council.

However, the view of our HEC and BBC informants was that fluoridation is a special case in that firstly, it is official DHSS policy to encourage health authorities to proceed with fluoridation[5] ; secondly, the scientific evidence for the efficacy of fluoridation in preventing dental caries is 'hard'; and thirdly, fluoridation of water supplies is a discrete social policy measure that does not threaten any major economic interests. In contrast, there is not as yet any national food policy; much of the scientific evidence relating to the aetiology and prevention of CHD is 'soft'; and most importantly, a government strategy for the prevention of CHD would, at the very least, pose a significant threat to the food and agricultural industries, and of course the tobacco industry, and (if the determinants of social inequalities in CHD were to be addressed) could ultimately have far reaching political and economic implications. This is not the kind of health education the HEC as a quango can easily be involved with.[6] To quote from an HEC officer:

I think there are bodies and organisations who can be more effective in the social policy area than [the HEC] can . . . campaigns like ASH for example [and] professional bodies — the Royal College of General Practitioners, and Royal College of Physicians, etc. — who are totally unrelated to government and they can say what they like on the basis of medical opinion and I think sometimes it is more appropriate that they do so, because of the very nature of the body that we are.

2. *The assumption that HEC publications should reflect a consensus of mainstream medical opinion*

We have described in Chapter 3 how the process of medical consultation for HEC publications is directed towards arriving at a consensus position that reflects mainstream medical opinion. This assumption that HEC publications should reflect a consensus of medical opinion again needs to be understood in the context of HEC's position as a DHSS-funded quango and the perceived political necessity to 'play safe'. *Beating Heart Disease* was described at an early stage of its production as:

> . . . a lovely illustration of [how] the advice that [HEC publications] give in the end turns out to be terribly bland because of having to play safe all the time.

However, this assumption also in part reflects:

> . . . the overall general wish to get the facts right and not to present the public with confusing or conflicting advice or advice that may change . . . we wanted it to be very much a practical booklet, we wanted to say to people 'look this is what most people think or what most doctors think, this is the gist of it, we will give you this advice . . . we are not absolutely 100 per cent sure but we are pretty confident it will help' . . .

3. *Assumptions about the information needs of the target audience*

The decision to focus on information that was practical in the sense of providing a 'consensus' of clear, straightforward guidelines for personal action, can be seen, in part, as a result of assumptions concerning the target audience of the booklet, and the amount of information suitable for such an audience. Central to such assumptions, is the almost universal and unquestioned dictate of health education that a publication targeted at 'the general public' (often, we have observed, a euphemistic reference to social classes IV and V) should be short and simple with a reading age no higher than that of a tabloid newspaper. Otherwise, it is argued, it will not be read. This underlies much of the critical feedback that the HEC receives from health education officers about its publications, and was a common theme of health education officers' replies to a Health Education Publications Project questionnaire about HEOs' criteria for evaluating health education publications. For example:

[they] must be simple and easy to read. Many leaflets have a readability that is far too high for the general public.

. . . leaflets which appear to be almost booklets with long texts and more complicated language are rarely of much use.

A lot of our customers are of limited intellectual ability and the need for brevity is consequently paramount.

[if] too detailed, not likely to be read. Reading level [must be] suitable for target audience — including social class considerations.

Assumptions about appropriate levels of information for health education publications, and the discrepancy between these assumptions and the perspective of the target audience, were a central area of investigation by the Health Education Publications Project. A detailed discussion of the findings has been presented elsewhere.[7] In brief, we would argue that the dictate that health education publications should be short and simple, although widespread, has little basis in research that has looked at information needs from a target audience perspective.[8] Instead, it can be seen as reflecting, in part at least, broader ideological perspectives of the professional middle classes;[9] and as being largely perpetuated, within health education, by methodological misconceptions — particularly concerning the nature, function and applicability of readability tests.[10]

Since *Beating Heart Disease* was to be distributed both to the general public through the usual HEO channels, and also in response to direct requests from Radio 4 listeners, 'pitching the information at an appropriate level' posed a dilemma for the HEC:

. . . we were rather torn between trying to get the level right for the radio series because it is meant to be in support of that chiefly, and then getting the level right for the rest of the world who would be reading it from then on . . .

The booklet, it was argued, had to be 'pretty simple stuff', but at the same time, could not be 'talking down' to Radio 4 listeners.

[there is] a problem in producing anything for an across-the-board, mass audience. If [the HEC] could split the booklet and have two booklets, one say *Daily Mirror, Sun, Star* level, and the other sort of somewhere between the *Express* and *Guardian,* in other words split them according to educational levels, then I think it could be quite reasonable and realistic to put down the various arguments [about CHD prevention] or to go into some of the arguments as to why there are differences of opinion . . . but when it comes to producing a simple booklet when all our research tells us that you have got to keep things clear and simple and straightforward otherwise people will not read it then you are up against it really, compromise again.

Inevitably, the final booklet did reflect a position of compromise both in terms of the tone and the amount of information presented. It was longer, more informative, and more detailed than is usual for HEC publications — a point that was picked up by the following HEO who commented on the draft text:

It [*Beating Heart Disease*] is very comprehensive, but does it meet the needs of the man on the street? . . . the ordinary person — not social classes I and II, but the ordinary mum with a husband who boozes too much . . .

However, as we discuss in Chapter 5, our pretesting of the booklet suggested that the amount of information still falls short of what representatives of the 'target audience' would have liked.

4. *The assumption that the HEC must 'sell health'*

The assumption that health education publications must be 'short and simple' and that they must not present the reader with 'conflicting or confusing advice' is integral to an approach that evaluates health education messages within an 'advertising'/'propagandist' framework. The overriding aim of the leaflet/poster implicit in many of the replies to the HEPP survey of health education officers' criteria for evaluating publications seemed to be: 'will it seduce, grab and attract the reader?' For example:

The main features of a good leaflet or poster must be simplicity, brevity, boldness of presentation, clarity and an 'arresting' style.

The prescriptive style of communication that is illustrated by *Beating Heart Disease*, whereby information is selectively presented to 'sell' a 'clear and simple' individualistic health education message can be traced to the propaganda function of pamphlets in the work of the HEC's predecessor, the Central Council for Health Education (1927-68).[11] The pressures for the HEC to continue to execute this propaganda function through its publications enterprise are illustrated by a *British Medical Journal* editorial published around the time of our research entitled 'New thoughts for the Health Education Council'.[12] The editorial stressed the need for the HEC to 'avoid those tedious arguments about whether the HEC is an educator or propagandist', adding 'undoubtedly it [the HEC] *must sell health*' (our italic).

Although, as already mentioned, *Beating Heart Disease* contained more information than is usual for HEC publications, it remained essentially prescriptive, with no attempt to enter into the arguments surrounding the areas of contention and dissension that are referred to in our discussion of the scientific evidence.

These then, were the sorts of general arguments that were used to justify both the individualistic orientation of *Beating Heart Disease* and its prescriptive communication style, whereby evaluation of the evidence relating the aetiology and prevention of CHD was taken out of the readers' hands. We shall now examine the problematic implications of the decision to focus on practical advice for individuals and of the assumptions underlying this decision, for the presentation of information in the booklet.

The problem of translating population data into practical advice for individuals

The decision to focus the booklet's message on the practicalities of what individuals could do for themselves meant that some of the more obvious political problems in relation to the HEC's role were avoided. But because (as indicated in Chapter 2) population data in support of a mass approach to prevention cannot readily be translated into individual advice, a new set of difficulties were created.

A number of comments on earlier drafts of the text from external consultants and from the HEC related to the questionable usefulness and/or validity of extrapolating from population data to the individual case. There was a general concern that the booklet:

> . . . seemed to be saying that this was how you could prevent heart disease when an individual can't necessarily prevent heart disease, they can only reduce the risk of getting it. There is no guarantee that if they did everything in the booklet then they would not have a heart attack; so [the HEC] had to change the emphasis.

The way in which the emphasis was changed was described to us as: 'by using lots of "it is likely that" and "may" and just not being definite', and by playing down the specific claims for the advice given in terms of prevention of CHD, at the same time as emphasizing the more general health benefits of following the advice. Thus the following introductory remarks in an earlier draft of the text: '. . . heart disease *can be beaten.* And it *can be prevented* if you know how' were replaced in the final draft by: '. . . you can do something *to reduce the risk.* And you'll not only be fighting heart disease. You'll soon feel fitter than ever before' (our italic).

Another example of use of wording to change the emphasis is where the phrase in an earlier draft: 'If there's a lot of fat in your diet you *are likely* to have a high level of cholesterol in your blood' was changed in the final draft to '. . . you *may* have a high level of cholesterol in your blood', after one consultant had commented that there is: '. . . very little evidence that *individuals* eating a lot of fat have higher blood cholesterol' (our italic). The rationale of this approach was explained to us as follows:

> When you've got a message with some degree of uncertainty I think you will have to be quite clear in your principles. In other words, if you are going to propose something like taking more exercise (as an example) there is absolutely no harm in being fairly positive about it — in other words you can say 'Take more exercise — it will probably do you some good, it certainly won't do you any harm' and I think therefore when you have an uncertainty, provided your message is positive and safe you don't have to be quite so rock solid in your evidence as if you are telling somebody 'Stop doing something' or to do something with some risks . . . Scientific information isn't all that hard in some cases. But I think you have to be reasonable . . . I think it is biological common sense that, for instance, adding exercise, or fibre to your diet, is likely to be beneficial and *not* likely to do harm. I would certainly push these things rather than some of the other more controversial things. I think you should pick out the positive ones. Stopping smoking — the evidence for this is good. Where you have good evidence, emphasize that.

There was also the problem of how to translate population data into specific practical advice that could be usefully tailored to the diverse individual needs of a heterogeneous target audience:

> . . . would you say to people you should cut salt intake down by one-third? . . . that's fine as a population, you want to see the population salt intake down by one-third, but who is to say that a particular individual isn't already low on salt? . . . Another might be taking tons of salt and should cut his salt intake down by three-quarters . . . it's the inherent problem of giving mass messages to people who are actually individuals.

Related to this, was the question of how to take account of the issue of multicausality in the presentation of lifestyle advice. Much of the early discussions about the format of the publication centred on various possibilities for grouping lifestyle factors, for example:

Yes, I had this trouble trying to work out which ones [risk factors] go with which. Certainly smoking and blood pressure are the big ones.

But it's not easy to pair them because smoking and blood pressure can be paired with diet of a sort, then we can also pair stress with blood pressure.

I was wondering whether you would put relaxation with blood pressure or exercise.

There are many different ways you can link them all up.

I mean perhaps we shouldn't link them, perhaps we should have them separate . . .

I would have thought you would probably have them as separate sections for each one really.

Can you just list them for me?

Yes. They are smoking, blood pressure, diet, . . . exercise, and then there is this question of stress — yes, personality. And you might want to do a separate section for women like the Pill, for instance, which should be given a mention . . .

Can we talk about smoking, diet, blood pressure and stress in [a] women's section?

The pragmatic solution that was finally adopted was acknowledged to be somewhat arbitrary and not perhaps the most helpful for readers:

It was very difficult to actually categorize factors, perhaps it was our fault in the first place for trying to treat heart disease like that by categorizing it 'things that can affect your heart', but we couldn't see any other way of doing it. Because they are all so interrelated I think that is perhaps where the booklet is a bit weak because it establishes false categories really, so that people might look at their health in relation to their heart in terms of different factors instead of trying to think about themselves as a whole. I think it was just an organizational difficulty really that led us to do that.

Case studies in the translation of scientific evidence: dietary goals and stress

1. *The dietary goals story*

The dietary goals story provides a clear illustration of the constraints imposed by the HEC's relationship with government.

The HEC's pragmatic solution to the problem referred to above, of translating population data into individual dietary advice, was to treat each reader as if they were eating the average British diet. Thus the draft text for *Beating Heart Disease* included the advice:

> . . . cut down on the total amount of fat you eat by *at least a quarter* . . .
> [and] cut down your intake [of saturated fat] *by half.* (our italic)

This information was based on the objectives for changes in the average British diet that were contained in a draft of the HEC programme for the prevention of CHD, which were in turn based on the population dietary guidelines contained in the report of the WHO Expert Committee on Prevention of CHD.[13]

However, just as *Beating Heart Disease* was about to go to print, it was made clear to the HEC that the DHSS did not accept the quantified dietary goals quoted in the draft HEC Programme. It was also made clear that the DHSS would object in the strongest possible terms to the publication of the objectives in their current quantified form, especially since a Committee (COMA) was being set up by the DHSS on this very subject. Reference was also made to the possibly adverse reaction of the Food Manufacturers' Foundation to such advice being published. The position that was consequently adopted in the final (1983/84) draft of the CHD Programme was that:

> Whilst it is recognized that, for the practical purpose of health education, there is a need to adopt more specific (i.e. quantified) behavioural objectives (for example with regard to dietary guidelines), before doing so the Council will await the outcome of three major developments in 1983-4 . . . [including] a report from the DHSS Committee on Medical Aspects of Food Policy which will consider the dietary aspects of heart disease.[14]

Although *Beating Heart Disease* was not itself subjected to DHSS scrutiny, the discussion about the CHD Programme had obvious implications for the booklet. The dilemma that confronted the HEC was described by one person as follows:

> . . . if [the HEC] simply erased the fixed quantified dietary goals and fol-
> lowed the line in *Eating for Health,* which is the government's own booklet,
> and just said simply reduce fats especially saturated fats, reduce sugar, reduce
> salt, and increase dietary fibre and complex carbohydrates without giving
> any figures or targets to aim at, then that might suffice . . . it would cer-
> tainly pacify or at least it would please the DHSS if [the HEC] did that,
> that is what they are asking [the HEC] to do. The only trouble is it would
> probably be considered by nutritionists and epidemiologists as lacking bite
> and being lacking of practical value.

The solution that was adopted was to change, for example, the quantified advice cited above to cutting down on total fat by '*up to* a quarter'
(instead of '*at least* a quarter'), and cutting down on saturated fats 'by
up to a half' (instead of '*by* half').

2.   *The stress story*

The HEC's handling of the issue of stress in relation to CHD highlights
the way in which information is steered towards a message that is both
medically and politically acceptable.

Internal HEC discussion documents that prepared the ground for the
Council's current Programme of Education for the Prevention of CHD
show that the link between stress and CHD was not denied by the HEC.
Furthermore, the HEC were not unaware that an effective strategy for
prevention of the adverse effects of stress requires intervention at more
than just an individual level. One of the objectives of an earlier draft of
the CHD Programme was:

> To increase public awareness of the possible links between so-called 'stress'
> and CHD [and] to encourage individual *and environmental* modifications
> to minimize adverse effects of stress (our italic).

By the final draft stage of the Programme, however, the wording of this
objective had been changed to:

> To increase public awareness of the putative link between certain parameters
> of so-called 'stress', high blood pressure, and CHD, and to promote tech-
> niques for avoiding or coping with such stress. However, the WHO Expert
> Committee noted that 'public and professional misconceptions about stress,
> whereby it is assigned a primary role in the genesis of CHD, may divert
> attention from demonstrated needs in prevention'.

The perceived need for the HEC to play down the role of social stress in the aetiology of CHD was explained to us as follows:

It is the most popular thing that people mention — stress — and the evidence for it is absolutely minimal. People love to explain things like heart disease on outside forces like pressures and stress and overwork and all the rest of it.

The same assumption about the need to correct public misconceptions about stress was evinced in an article in *Health Education News* in 1981 entitled 'Heart disease risks ignored'.[15] The article presents results from an HEC-commissioned market research survey on public attitudes to CHD which it reports as showing that:

53 per cent of Britons believe stress to be the major cause of heart attacks [even though] stress is not currently recognized as a medical condition.

The article goes on to quote Dr Keith Taylor, (then HEC Director General Designate) as commenting:

The results of this survey show that most of the public do not know what are the important risk factors for developing a heart attack.

This article was subsequently cited as a major source of evidence of the 'inadequate understanding of the "causes" of heart disease on the part of the [British] public'.[16] The HEC publicity files contained cuttings from over twenty newspapers reporting on the *Health Education News* article carrying headings such as 'Ignorance about the big killer disease'; 'Most people unaware of heart risks'; 'Heart attack ignorance highlighted by survey'. The article was also reported in scientific journals, such as the *New Scientist* and the *Lancet*.

Contrary to the impression conveyed by the publicity about the HEC survey, the evidence that we have cited in Chapter 2 of this paper would suggest that the fact that '53 per cent of Britons believe stress to be the major cause of heart attacks' does not necessarily constitute evidence of an inadequate understanding of the causes of CHD. Manicom,[17] in a subsequent issue of *Health Education News,* reviewed some of the literature hypothesizing stress as a major linking factor between an individual's physical well-being, and his or her psychosocial environment and concluded that:

The public may have a more sophisticated understanding of the causes of disease than the medical profession.

The HEC policy of countering the importance that the public attach to stress in the aetiology of CHD was reflected in the drafting of *Beating Heart Disease*. For example, the section of the booklet entitled 'Is stress bad for the heart?' was introduced in an earlier draft of the text, by the paragraph.

> Most people would put stress at the top of their list of things that are bad for the heart. It seems obvious that worry and anxiety, or frequent crises and rows, can make your blood pressure go up and lead to a heart attack. *But there is still very little scientific evidence to prove this,* partly because stress is almost impossible to measure and define. (our italic)

This double standard in the publication's treatment of the status of scientific evidence relating to stress, as compared with other lifestyle factors, was questioned by one of the professional consultants who pointed out that the scientific evidence for many of the other statements in the publication was 'little if any stronger'. The final sentence of the paragraph just quoted was subsequently changed to:

> But *this is still difficult to prove,* partly because stress is almost impossible to measure and define. (our italic)

This paragraph is then followed by a section entitled 'How you can cope with stress' which briefly acknowledges the presence of stress related factors outside an individual's control, but then focuses on some techniques (deep breathing, clench-and-let-go exercises, meditation and general exercise) for coping with the effects of stress at an individual level. Here, as elsewhere in the booklet, the role of the social environment is understated, whilst the individual as a target for behaviour change or adaptation is emphasized. The available evidence was selectively presented to support a strategy of health education for individual change.

Chapter 5

Lay Perspectives on
Beating Heart Disease

> The process of educational osmosis is unidirectional, with information pass-
> ing from the scientific community to the lay public . . . By contrast, relatively
> little is known by the scientific community about lay theories concerning
> [health-related behaviour] and particularly, about their susceptibility to
> modification and change in response to 'scientific fact'.[1]

> . . . health education specialists proceed as if they were pouring their ideas
> and appeals into a void instead of an existing popular health culture.[2]

There is now an increased recognition, in theory at least, of the value,
and indeed necessity, for health education of exploring and giving credibility to lay health beliefs. For example, the HEC Health Education Studies
Unit in their final report on the Patient Project,[3] conclude that:

> To be understood and accepted . . . health education needs to relate to the
> sense people make of their personal experience . . . We suggest in fact that
> [lay] beliefs are a potentially rich resource for achieving much higher levels
> of understanding of health issues, including the need for prevention and
> anticipatory care, provided they are seriously explored.

Research which has taken as its starting point the health experiences
and concerns of the lay public, has provided rich data on the depth and
complexity of lay knowledge, beliefs and values regarding the causation
and prevention of ill-health; on the extent of match and mismatch between this lay perspective and the assumptions underlying the traditional
approach to health education; and on the implication of health educators'
failure to take account of this lay perspective for the outcome of health
education campaigns.[4] That health education messages should evolve
from people's expressed information needs and experiences is the central
argument of a community development approach to health education, a

style of working that is receiving increasing acceptance and recognition as a way forward.[5]

In Chapter 3 we described the production process of *Beating Heart Disease* and drew attention to the lack of meaningful input, at any stage of production, from the target audience — i.e. the general public. We described how, instead, judgements were made about the target audience and what information was 'best' for them. In this chapter we shall explore lay health beliefs about CHD aetiology and prevention, using some qualitative data from our pretesting of *Beating Heart Disease* by way of illustration. We have structured the chapter around major themes emerging from the pretesting data, namely, the lay assessment and balancing of risk, and particularly the way in which people see their health problems and the potential for individual prevention as deeply embedded in the social and economic fabric of their everyday lives; the wish for more information than *Beating Heart Disease* provided; the wish for more discussion of the lack of consensus and of the uncertainties in the scientific evidence, and finally, the rejection of the prescriptive propagandist style of the health education message. We shall use representative quotes from our data to illustrate these themes, and, where possible, supplement our pretesting data with a discussion of other research work on lay health beliefs that has identified similar themes.

The pretesting data presented is drawn from hypothesis-generating material from in-depth, semi-structured interviews that we conducted with 21 adults — 12 women and 9 men — ranging in age from 16 to 61, with approximately an equal number of working-class and middle-class people. Further details of the sample and of the research design and methodology are presented in the report submitted to the HEC.[6]

For the purpose of pretesting, the designers of *Beating Heart Disease* produced a colour mock-up of a three-page spread from the booklet, which covered an introduction to 'what causes heart disease' and sections on 'smoking' and 'bad eating habits'. These sections essentially contained and reflected the general health education message of the booklet. They also contained a representation of the design used throughout. After respondents had been given a chance to study the three-page spread in detail, they were asked for their general and specific reactions to the content and the design, their views on the aetiology and prevention of CHD, and on the preventive message of *Beating Heart Disease*, and their general views about health education publications. To supplement the individual interviews, we also arranged a group discussion with eight 15/16 year olds, structured around similar questions. The data from this group discussion is not presented here; it produced similar themes, however, to those discussed in this chapter.

Lay perspectives on CHD aetiology and prevention

In the last chapter we discussed how the HEC, in translating current knowledge about CHD aetiology and prevention, selectively presented information to support an individualistic health education message that focused on practical advice for individuals. We explained how in doing this, the lack of hard evidence to support much of the individual advice in the booklet was glossed over, the role of the wider socio-economic environment was largely ignored and epidemiological evidence implicating social and economic factors in the aetiology of CHD was played down. Although the HEC were careful in the main text of the booklet to avoid making unsubstantiated claims about the potential of individual behaviour change for preventing CHD, the general prescriptive tone of the booklet tended to foster a different impression — one of a direct causal relationship between smoking, diet and CHD. Furthermore, in the absence of any explanation of the probabilistic nature of the association between risk factors and disease manifestation, of the difference between a population's and an individual's risk, and of the difficulty of translating population data into individual advice, the perceived medical contention that smoking *causes* CHD, for example, seemed to be dismissed by the following respondents because of contrasting personal 'proof':

> This smoking lark — I don't believe it. I buried my uncle yesterday. He and my auntie both had valves fitted. My auntie smokes like a trooper, and he didn't smoke at all, and yet his body rejected the valve and she's carried on fine.

> There are people in their nineties who smoked all their life, and are overweight, and as fit as a fiddle.

These kind of quotes are often cited by health professionals as illustrations of lay ignorance of orthodox medical 'facts' about disease aetiology, and of the need to correct this ignorance through health education. The findings from our pretesting were consistent with those of Graham [7] who, in a paper on 'Smoking in pregnancy: The attitudes of expectant mothers' shows that it is not ignorance of 'the facts' so much as the credibility the individual accords to these facts, as presented in health education literature, *vis-à-vis* personal 'proof' that has been built up over years of observation and experience.

In Chapter 4 we made reference to the HEC's worries that the structure of *Beating Heart Disease* established 'false categories' in its presentation of the risk factors. The quotes presented below illustrate the ways in which our respondents seemed not to think of risks as discrete entities, each to be considered separately, but rather seemed to balance 'risks' against one another. In this sense, these quotes suggested that people assess the relative significance of risks within the complexities of their everyday lives:

He [my son] stopped smoking, but started again because he put on weight.

My husband says that if he gives up the pipe he would be more stressed without it, so what can you do?

Everyone knows smoking damages your health . . . it doesn't bother me that I smoke. It did when I was on the pill and had high blood pressure.

My wife's a nurse and she smokes like a trooper. She accepts it as a possible risk . . . the pressures of mental hospital work and social reinforcement — the patients smoke, and the nurses . . . and coming to terms with the possibility of dying. [his wife had undergone treatment for cancer of the womb]

I think [smoking] does pull you down but when you've got three kids running around the house it's ridiculous trying to stop.

What these quotes also suggest is that some 'unhealthy behaviours' are seen as 'healthier' than others, in both a physical and mental sense. Hilary Graham, in recent research conducted for the HEC, has provided survey data on how mothers 'cope' on a day-to-day basis with caring for pre-school children which supports this theme. Her data suggests that:

activities which seemingly threaten *individual* health may play a significant part in the maintenance of *family* health. The prime example here is smoking . . . The evidence from the smokers suggests that smoking provided a way of structuring and managing daily life: the majority of smokers noted that they smoked in response to particular situations and the majority felt that smoking helped them cope with their day-to-day responsibilities.[8]

The responses from our pretesting on the balancing of health risks can also be seen as lending support to other research findings that have suggested the need to question the assumption that health, in the narrow disease-related sense, is equally salient for everyone. For example, a Social Science Research Council survey designed to elicit respondents' own definitions of 'quality of life' found that health was awarded a relatively low priority, compared to such things as family, home life, marriage, general contentment, money and prices, and also standard of living or decent conditions of life. Similarly, before the launch of its 'Look After Yourself!' (LAY) campaign in 1977, the HEC commissioned some market research on public attitudes to the concept of a 'Better Health Guide', which would give advice on diet, exercise, smoking and stress to help individuals lead a healthier and longer life. The reaction of respondents to the idea of the 'Better Health Guide' were in many respects very similar to the reactions that we record here to *Beating Heart Disease*, i.e. the lack of importance attached to living a longer and healthier life in relation to other quality of life priorities.[9] The following quotes illustrate further the context in which respondents evaluated health risks as they were presented to them in *Beating Heart Disease*:

> . . . will people take notice of that? . . . If ordinary people read this and see they have to keep their weight down and stop smoking, there's nothing to live for . . .

> My husband was on a 2000 calorie diet [before he died of heart disease] . . . salad — it takes all the pleasure out of living . . . better to live a shorter life.

> Butter's the main part of your life. What's a chip butty without the butter?

> I prefer to be slightly overweight — you don't get knocked over at rugby so much.

> Why make life miserable? You might as well have a shorter and happier life.

It would seem essential that health education considers the implications of this emerging picture of lay risk-assessment and salience of physical health, for the way it structures health information and advice.

Perhaps the most significant theme to emerge from the pretesting data in relation to lay health beliefs on CHD aetiology and general disease causation, was the way in which respondents saw their health problems as deeply embedded in the social and economic fabric of their everyday lives. When we asked what respondents considered to be the major causes of CHD, their answers suggested that whilst, in the main, they did not deny that smoking, diet and blood pressure have some part to play in the aetiology of CHD, they saw these factors as only part of the story. Furthermore, their responses suggested that they see disease aetiology as not necessarily specific to one disease, and their responses consequently seemed to focus more on the main causes of *disease* generally and not just the causes of CHD. The following quotes provide a flavour of the way respondents perceived disease aetiology:

> It's always smoking . . . they're always the same these things in books — they always go into smoking in detail, nothing else. There are bound to be other causes — but they say a bit about that and then have pages and pages about smoking.

> Smoking can be injurious to the heart but that's not 100 per cent to blame. I worked for a chemical firm and used to line tins [for food] . . . The preservatives and things that go into food. You're not eating uncontaminated food. Even the food from the garden is sprayed with insecticides.

> Smelly jobs — like steel workers and asbestos factories give you cancer — and heart disease?

> There's chemicals in the ground now. Everything's false grown . . . then again, all the stuff from fumes, greater danger really than smoking.

> Stress, worrying about a job, whether you're going to be able to pay the mortgage, keep the family.

> . . . it's a lot to do with worry — if a woman has a husband out of work — unemployment means people have a lot of stress and worry . . . This time is more worrying than others, and it creates lots of illness.

> . . . stress and the pace we live at in the Western world — the way we live, the pace we live at. You're just picking out two things — smoking and food . . . [other causes are] the rate at which we do things, the pressure our system puts on us, the way we live — work harder to get money, buy more things, and it goes on and on . . . overworking your body.

These quotes need to be interpreted in the context of recent epidemiological and psychosocial research (discussed in Chapter 2) that is looking to the wider social and economic environment, and at the significance of chronic social stress, as a way of understanding the social distribution of CHD and of other major causes of ill-health in our society. It is interesting also to contrast the quotes on the role of stress with the HEC's handling of the issue of stress, discussed in Chapter 4, where the HEC attempted to play down social stress as an aetiological factor in CHD (in accordance with WHO guidelines).

The lay model of disease aetiology suggested above is consistent with findings from other research that has been concerned with identifying health priorities from a lay perspective. Common health concerns that have been identified by community health projects and surveys include the health implications of poverty, inadequate housing, environmental pollution, lack of open space, social isolation, lack of child-care facilities, and the pervasive stresses associated with occupying an underprivileged position within a socially stratified society.[10]

Lay concerns about the possibilities for individual prevention
In the introduction to this paper and the previous chapter we discussed how *Beating Heart Disease* epitomizes the individual behaviour-change model of health education, which has increasingly been the subject of much criticism, both for its 'victim-blaming' implications and, related to this, its apparent assumptions that individuals, if motivated, will be in a position to change their behaviour. The following respondents had clearly internalized this victim-blaming ideology:

A lot is spent [by the NHS] on treating stupid people [for heart disease].

A lot of women, when the children go, are inclined to spoil the man. They can kill a man with kindness, they can. Later on in life a woman gives a man what he fancies. She has no intention to give him a heart attack, just to please him.

Others (though still seeing the individual as the problem for change) hinted at being unconvinced by the possibilities for individual behaviour-oriented health education:

. . . bad living . . . I don't know how you make people change the way they live — they probably know that but don't change.

. . . it's hard to make people change their life-styles — it's fine for you and I, but . . .

The majority of respondents, however, cited examples of the very real constraints that people experience at both the macro and the micro level in attempting to reduce their risk of ill-health through behavioural change.

On the macro level of analysis, several respondents talked about the constraints of living in a society where health pursuits are essentially in conflict with economic interests. The following quote illustrates the type of response to a question on whether there is anything the government could do to reduce the risk of CHD:

> I don't think for one minute government will do anything to assist in help-ing with tobacco or drinking with the revenue they get from it. If they can get money they don't give a damn if they kill you in the process. As long as they get the pound out of your pocket.

The need for *Beating Heart Disease* to acknowledge such macro-constraints, rather than serve the illusion that we *as individuals* can con-trol our own health, was mentioned by one respondent:

> [it] should avoid attaching individual blame but that's what it's all about — how to change your habits . . . it could talk about smoking, diet, etc, but it should also talk about the reasons why people eat bad diets and smoke — like the government's interest in perpetuating bad health by their interest in tax from tobacco sales.

Turning to a micro level of analysis, the quotes below illustrate the con-straints of money and time in trying to follow a healthy diet, constraints documented by other researchers and mentioned by several of our respondents:

> If you work you have to have convenience foods — you won't come home and start cooking unless you're very organized and do it the night before or in the morning. It's a time thing — how much time you have left.

> This thing with food would cost you a fortune! I buy cheaper cuts of meat that are fattier. Chicken costs more . . . My mother had a big family — eleven of us. We were brought up on belly pork — that's the cheapest you can get . . . I cook like my mother cooked . . . There's no choice nowadays. The cheaper cuts of meat are always the fattier cuts.

Another key theme to emerge in respondents' discussion of the constraints they experienced was the issue of who controls food eaten in the home. A crucial target audience for *Beating Heart Disease* was described by the HEC as 'probably . . . in most cases the spouse of the bloke who is likely to get a heart attack'. This assumption is reflected in the booklet in the section on diet by the sentence 'And if you are choosing food for the family, you've got their hearts in your hands too'. In this way, the booklet reflects a prevailing health education ideology that sees women as responsible for reducing risk in family lifestyle, implying that as wives, and as mothers, women are in a position to control not only their own but other's diets. Whilst the women we talked to showed very clearly how they had internalized this responsibility, it was clear that they didn't, in fact, have control over what other members of the family ate:

> I try and give them a good staple diet. If they like fresh vegetables you're on a winner, but you can't force them to eat it. I choose what we all like. If one doesn't like something then four of us don't have it . . . They wouldn't like the high fibre. I've tried and they don't like it so I don't see why they should have to eat it.

> I try and cut down his potatoes . . . I don't tell him, but he gets up from the table and eats bread instead.

> He's always eating chips and has acne spots — I try and tell him it's his diet but I may as well hit my head against a brick wall.

> She [my mother] gives me what I like. *Q:* What would you do if she served you the kind of food recommended in the booklet? Not eat it. Go and buy myself chips and a pie.

One respondent pointed out that the HEC booklet also ignores the fact that not all food is eaten within the home:

> . . . it assumes the person who chooses the food — the mother — is totally responsible for bad eating habits, but its not showing how school food is a problem or canteen food, or just the sort of food that's available.

The significance of who controls food eaten in the home and the implications for health education have been discussed in detail elsewhere.[12]

Lay evaluation of the level of information and the prescriptive strategy of health education
In the context of the lay perspectives on CHD aetiology and prevention presented above, we now move on to look briefly at how the amount and style of information in *Beating Heart Disease* was evaluated. We shall suggest that the assumptions made by the HEC about the information needs of the target audience and about the role of HEC publications (see

Chapter 4) were in fact unfounded, and ultimately could prevent the booklet's aims and objectives from being met.

Earlier in this paper (Chapter 4) we discussed the assumptions, so prevalent in health education, about appropriate levels of information for publications. We also mentioned how, because *Beating Heart Disease* was specifically targeted at a Radio 4 audience as well as at the general public, it was somewhat more informative and detailed than is usual for HEC publications. Nevertheless, findings suggest that far from being pitched at too high a level, as the HEC feared, information needs of the respondents were inadequately met. We asked respondents the summary question of whether they thought, on balance, the amount of information contained in the booklet was about right, too much or too little. Speaking for themselves,[13] no one thought there was too much information, and about half of those asked thought there was too little (with similar responses for middle-class and working-class respondents). Common reactions to the general message of the booklet were:

It contains nothing I didn't know already and nothing that the majority of the public don't know.

A lot of it is common knowledge; could be more detail, more explanation.

It didn't go into sufficient depth.

Specifically, respondents would have liked more information in terms of understanding, and in being able to evaluate and make use personally of the advice given:

The link between fat and heart disease is not explained very well.

. . . more on the anatomy and physiology side — about the effects of smoking, etc.

. . . what saturated and unsaturated fats are.

Why is the risk greater if you're over 35 and on the pill?

. . . more in terms of giving variety, e.g. for fat people. It's not their fault they need different advice than someone who's thin. This only caters for the average — someone about my size.

As far as eating's concerned it's not very explanatory on (different dietary requirements for) different jobs, it could be a bit more explanatory.

You should give variety. We're all individuals, we all think differently. Could put more in on the food angle, could say if you're not going to eat this — because some people won't have the choice — then at least list the best of the worst.

It seems, then, that the worries of the authors of *Beating Heart Disease* (referred to in Chapter 4) about giving 'mass messages to people who are actually individuals' and the continual compromises resulting in blandness, were reflected in respondents' evaluation of the booklet. It also seems that the effect of pitching the information in *Beating Heart Disease* at a 'pretty simple' level was to leave respondents feeling uninformed on many of the issues of the CHD debate, and feeling that they lacked the detailed information required to relate practical advice to their own personal situation.

The hypothesis that professional health educators tend to underestimate the information needs of 'ordinary' readers of health education publications, suggested by the pretesting data presented here, is supported by research by the Health Education Publications Project which involved a comparison of lay and professional reactions to a 120-page draft text of a menopause publication, that had been developed in response to the expressed information needs of women of menopause age. Professionals were significantly more likely than women of menopause age to consider that the amount of information in the booklet was 'too much'. Furthermore, this research — in keeping with the findings of other research that has investigated health information needs from a consumer perspective — did not provide any support for the professional assumption that working-class people want less health information than middle-class people. Researchers at the Centre for Mass Communications Research, Leicester, evaluating the HEC Education for Pregnancy and Parenthood Programme, have similarly identified a discrepancy between lay and professional perceptions of appropriate levels of information for health education publications aimed at 'ordinary' people.[15]

In the previous chapter we showed how and why the HEC made a decision not to enter into discussion of the areas of inconclusiveness, uncertainty and inconsistency in the scientific evidence relating to the aetiology and prevention of CHD. Yet, our interviews with respondents suggested that they were only too aware of the sometimes equivocal nature of 'expert' knowledge and that by not acknowledging this, the HEC might, in fact, be presenting a *more* confusing and *less* credible message:

They [expert] all say different things, don't they? . . . diet for instance. On the radio you hear potatoes are good for you and bread is good for you, and then you read, 'No, you put on weight'. You don't know who to believe.

You read one thing about diet and then it's all changed the next (e.g. baked beans). I tended to feel guilty each time I had some, now it's all changed, they're good for you.

I'm not convinced so much about the butter and fat thing now. There's been a bit of a rethink over the last year. The thinking about butter is rather hypothetical at the moment.

These quotes illustrate the high level of cynicism expressed by some respondents in their reactions to the style of information in *Beating Heart Disease*, cynicism based on the contrast between the authoritative tone of the booklet and their own evaluation of the status of 'expert knowledge'. One respondent suggested to us:

It turns me off that phrase [in text of booklet] 'take the expert's advice' . . . I don't like the use of the term 'expert' — it makes whatever comes after it sound authoritative and right, and that's misleading.

We would argue that the effect of the selective presentation of scientific evidence to support a consensus position, far from avoiding confusion, was to confuse respondents still further, to undermine the credibility of 'experts' and to obscure the distinction between health education originating from a 'neutral' organization and that put out by commercial vested interests. As a *Lancet*[16] editorial on CHD observed:

Ignoring apparently awkward findings is likely, in the long run, to be as harmful as overinterpreting those that seem to fit. Both undermine the general credibility of those from whom advice may be sought.

Cynicism was also apparent in reactions to the case history photo and caption on smoking that respondents were shown. They were well aware of how information can be manipulated to make a point:

Case histories don't have much impact unless you know the person. You get so many photos like that with quotes and you can't guarantee that's what any said. It's like all this stuff on TV with people saying 'I had to write to you about how white my washing is — can I now have my cheque please?'

[Case studies are useful] only if it's someone famous who you recognize or can put a name to. He's just an ordinary man walking down the street. He could be anyone — for all you know he might sit down after saying that and have a cigarette.

They're all the same . . . they always say that as if they've been given it to say, . . . told: 'Here's some money so say this for our book', it's always the same old thing.

In this sense, then, it seems that the HEC booklet was seen as using case-histories (a major design feature of the publication) in the same way as advertisers — to *sell* a point (or product):

. . . if you use it [the case history] to piece together an argument and explain that there's a range of experience and opinion then it's OK, but if you use it to prove a point then it's misleading.

The reactions of our respondents would seem to lend support to McCron's argument that:

Health campaigns using [a] commercial model tend to be regarded by people . . . as advertising, and hence . . . the information contained in them is open to suspicion.[17]

On philosophical grounds alone we would argue that it is neither ethical nor intellectually honest for the HEC, as the major official body disseminating preventive health information in this country, to perpetuate the notion that health is a product, or a commodity, that can be 'packaged' and 'sold' by health education, as distinct from an integral part of human life that is deeply embedded in the social and economic fabric of society. However, even leaving such arguments aside, the findings discussed here suggest that, ultimately, 'selling' a predefined message in *Beating Heart Disease* does not work and might have longer-term implications in terms of turning people off future health education messages.

The end result of a majority of respondents' evaluation of the information in *Beating Heart Disease* was a weariness about, and rejection of, 'the same old message':

Nothing new.

It's the same as everyone says . . . it goes on and on.

We just put it aside.

Chapter 6
Conclusions

The 'rules' of coronary prevention have, it seems, become an accepted wisdom of the 1980s. By smoking, eating too much of the wrong food and not getting enough exercise and relaxation, we as individuals, are indulging in risky living, and we must aim to modify our unhealthy behaviours. The HEC publication *Beating Heart Disease* presents and reflects these established guidelines for CHD prevention to a mass audience, and has been accompanied by advice from the DHSS,[1] regional and district health authority initiatives on CHD prevention,[2] and a wide range of exhortations, advice and information in the media. Not only have the guidelines for CHD prevention been increasingly presented as axiomatic, but so too has the discourse within which such guidelines are placed. A consensus of opinion on the role of the conventional 'risk factors' in the aetiology of CHD is suggested, and, from such consensus, the justification for prescriptive advice-giving flows. CHD aetiology and its prevention have, it seems, been rendered unproblematic in their theoretical base.

In this paper we have used the production of *Beating Heart Disease* as a case-study in the politics of health information and health education, and have attempted to 'tell the story' around the creation of this particular set of guidelines.

In Chapter 2 we discussed the scope of scientific evidence in relation to CHD aetiology and prevention. We argued that the current state of knowledge about CHD is far from unproblematic, and we highlighted ways in which the current CHD debate illustrates salient features in the social construction of knowledge. We discussed how the vested interests of the food and tobacco industry, government and the medical profession can all be seen to contribute to a particular individualistic, behaviour-oriented view of CHD and health education. In this sense, we argued, such interests serve an ideological purpose in reinforcing the values of conventional health education and, at the same time, diverting attention away from a different model of CHD aetiology and prevention — one that is more threatening to medical and political orthodoxies.

In Chapter 2 we also attempted to point out the contribution that a social perspective can, and we believe should, properly make to the CHD debate. Indeed, Linnie Price[3] argues that to ignore the evidence that social factors are important in the aetiology of CHD, is to imply that CHD is 'a phenomenon which operates independently of social factors'. We hope to have shown in this paper that neither in the findings of epidemiological research (Chapter 2) nor in the minds and everyday lives of ordinary people (Chapter 5) does CHD 'operate independently of social factors'. CHD and its prevention must inevitably be firmly embedded within the social and economic fabric of everyday lives.

The critique of conventional health education (Chapters 3 and 4) is now a well established one. The conventional health education approach to CHD prevention, as reflected in the production of *Beating Heart Disease* (Chapters 3 and 4), can be seen as victim-blaming and individualistic in its orientation, dogmatic and prescriptive in its 'top-down' approach and consensus-presenting concerns. It encourages a view of CHD that ignores or minimizes the role of the social environment in which individuals live, and thereby, ultimately reduces health education's own chances of effectiveness.

In supporting a social perspective, we are not denying the importance of individuals as actors in CHD prevention, or as recipients of health information, but rather are calling for a style of health education that is more intellectually honest in its reflection of epidemiological evidence, and more sensitive, appropriate and empowering to the lives of the individuals it addresses. We have suggested, here and elsewhere, [4] the need for health education to integrate, more fully than happens at present, theories of community development into the everyday practice of health education.

Can the HEC and health education generally, develop a style of working that enables the ideas and suggestions being offered here realistically to inform their everyday practice? We have been concerned throughout the writing of this paper to help the reader understand, and make sense of, the very real constraints under which the HEC (and by implication, state-funded health education) operates. We hope not to have underestimated or misrepresented the structural and ideological constraints, and hence to have been guilty of the very 'victim-blaming' we ourselves condemn. An HEC representative, in commenting on an earlier draft of this paper, suggested to us 'the political impossibility, at the current time, of the HEC being able to be intellectually more honest', in terms of its position as an organization whose role is increasingly seen by the government as one of disseminating an official ideology of health. At the same time it has been suggested to us that:

> it is to the discredit of our message that we get constrained, either by government or by commercial bodies. The great strength of the HEC should be that it is seen as only interested in providing a health message. It should not be constrained by government views and it should not be constrained by commercial interests . . . When it gets embroiled and either ends up being bought off by companies or being seen as the government's mouthpiece, some sort of government health propaganda, [the HEC] will lose credibility.

We have documented elsewhere[5] a number of recent examples of good practice in the production of HEC publications which indicate, albeit in a limited way, an increased willingness to question some of the traditional assumptions and values of the publications production process that have been the subject of criticism in this paper. We have cited isolated examples of the HEC's being prepared to challenge the myth of political neutrality on health issues and to take a stand against Government pressure to put 'wealth before health'. We have also noted the increased recognition by the HEC of the importance of taking account of lay perspectives and beliefs if health education is to connect effectively with the lives of its 'target audience'.

We want to end by quoting from the World Health Organization European Region's 'Health for All by the Year 2000' strategy document[6] which, we believe, provides a possible framework and legitimation for the HEC and health education generally, to challenge the political ideology and medical paradigm in which they are located.

> It is people who ultimately decide on the value of health in their lives, although their real options may be severely restricted by the economic, social, cultural and physical environment . . . People have the right to be informed . . . Collectively [health professionals] share the responsibility for broadening the framework traditionally used to define and analyse health problems, by looking more into the psychological, social, economic and environmental determinants of health . . . and stressing the importance of acting on those determinants if health is to be improved. Health professionals should also help in making the facts in this regard better known to the public . . .

Notes and References

Preface

1. Farrant, W, and Russell, J. (1985), *Health Education Council Publications: a case study in the production, distribution and use of health information,* Health Education Publications Project, University of London Institute of Education. To be published 1987 by National Extension College, Cambridge.

Chapter 1

1. Tuckett, D. (1979), 'Choices for health education: a sociological view' in I. Sutherland (ed.), *Health Education: Perspectives and Choices.* George Allen & Unwin, London.

2. Farrant and Russell (1985), op.cit. Preface above.

3. See for example: McKinlay, J.B. (1974), 'A case for refocusing upstream: the political economy of illness', *Behavioural Science Data Review,* June; Crawford, R. (1977), 'You are dangerous to your health: the ideology and politics of victim-blaming', *International Journal of Health Services,* Vol.7; Brown, E.R., Margo, G.E. (1978), 'Health education: can the reformers be reformed?' *International Journal of Health Services,* Vol.8; Freudenberg, N. (1978), 'Shaping the future of health education from behaviour change to social change', *Health Education Monographs,* Vol.6, No.4; Doyal, L. (1979), *The Political Economy of Health.* Pluto Press, London; Holtzman, N. (1979), 'Prevention: rhetoric and reality', *International Journal of Health Services,* Vol.9; Tuckett (1979), op.cit. n.1 above; Draper, P., Griffiths, J., Dennis, J. and Popay, J. (1980), 'Three types of health education', *British Medical Journal,* Vol.1, pp.493-5; Cornwell, J. (1984), *Hard-earned Lives: accounts of health and illness from East London.* Tavistock, London. Graham, H. (1984), *Women, Health and the Family.* Wheatsheaf Books, Brighton; Mitchell, J. (1984), *What Is To Be Done about Illness and Health?* Penguin Books, Harmondsworth; Kenner, C. (1985), *No Time for Women.* Pandora Press, London.

4. Marmot, M.G. (1986), 'Epidemiology and the art of the soluble', *Lancet,* 19 April, pp.897-900.

5. Beattie, A. (1984), 'Evaluating community health initiatives' in *Papers from the Conference 'Community Development in Health: addressing the confusions'* held at the King's Fund Centre, 13 June. An 'appraising institutional agendas' approach to evaluation is described by Beattie as one 'which seeks to identify and map as widely as possible the "context" — social, cultural, political — within which a particular programme is conducted. . . . This approach has its foundations in policy studies and political sciences, and draws upon the disciplines of social history and cultural anthropology.' Beattie describes an 'analysing clients' perspectives' approach to evaluation as one: 'which has gathered momentum recently and which aims to elicit and/or articulate the reactions of clients to particular social interventions. . . . Such techniques. . . . have been brought to prominence in the health field most especially in connection with studies of women's experience of health care and health education.'

Chapter 2

1. Department of Health and Social Security (1981), *Prevention and Health: avoiding heart attacks.* HMSO, London.

2. Open University (1985), *Health and Disease* U205 Book 8: Dilemmas and Prospects. Open University, Milton Keynes.

3. Oliver, M.F. (1982), 'Does control of risk factors prevent coronary heart disease?' *British Medical Journal,* Vol. 285, pp.1065-66

4. *The Times Health Supplement* (1982), 'Curbing a killer'.

5. Bartley, M. (1985), in 'CHD and the public health 1850-1983', *Sociology of Health and Illness,* Vol.7, No.3, pp.289-313, takes this further, suggesting that the disease category 'CHD' can itself be seen as socially constructed.

6. *Lancet* (1983), 'Diet and ischaemic heart disease — agreement or not?' 6 August, Vol.2, pp.317-19.

7. See, for example, the British Cardiac Society and Royal College of Physicians report on CHD prevention, 1976; WHO Expert Committee (1982), *Prevention of Coronary Heart Disease,* Technical Report Series No.678. World Health Organization, Geneva; Health Education Council (1984), *CHD Prevention: plans for action,* Pitman, London; and WHO Expert Committee (1986), *Community Prevention and Control of Cardiovascular Diseases,* Technical Report Series No.732. World Health Organization, Geneva.

8. Lewis, B. et. al. (1986), 'Reducing the risks of CHD in Individuals and in the population', *Lancet.* 26 April, pp.956-9.

9. Marmot, M. (1984), 'Lifestyle and national and international trends in CHD mortality', *Postgraduate Medical Journal,* Vol. 60, pp.3-8.

10. Morris, J.N., Marr, J.W., Heady, J.A., Mills, G.L. and Pilkington, T.R.E. (1963), 'Diet and plasma cholesterol in 99 bankmen', *British Medical Journal,* Vol. 1, pp.571-6; WHO Expert Committee (1982), op.cit. n.7 above.

11. For example see Guberan, E. (1979), 'Surprising decline of cardiovascular mortality in Switzerland: 1951-1976', *Journal of Epidemiology and Community Health,* Vol.33, pp.114-20; *Lancet* (1980), 'Why the American decline in coronary heart disease?' Vol.1, pp.183-4; Marmot (1984), op.cit. n.9 above.

12. See for example, Welin, L., Larsson, B., Svardsudd, K., and Wilhelmsen, L. (1983), 'Why is the incidence of ischaemic heart disease in Sweden increasing?: study of men born in 1913 and 1923', *Lancet,* 14 May, pp.1087-9.

13. St George, D.P. (1983), 'Is coronary heart disease caused by an environmentally-induced chronic metabolic imbalance?' *Medical Hypotheses,* Vol.12, pp.283-96.

14. Committee on Medical Aspects of Food Policy (1984), *Diet and Cardiovascular Disease.* Department of Health and Social Security, London.

15. Le Fanu, J. (1983), 'An end to a '70s dream', *Medical News,* 26 May.

16. Marmot, M.G. and Winkelstein, W. (1975), 'Epidemiologic observations on intervention trials for the prevention of CHD', *American Journal of Epidemiology.* Vol.101, No.3, pp.177-81.

17. Townsend, P. and Davidson, N. (eds.) (1982), *Inequalities in Health: the Black Report.* Penguin, Harmondsworth.

18. Marmot, M.G., Rose, G., Shipley, M. and Hamilton, P.J.S. (1978), 'Employment grade and coronary heart disease in British civil servants', *Journal of Epidemiology and Community Health,* Vol.32, pp.244-9.

19. Marmot, M.G., Rose, G. and Shipley, M.J. (1984), 'Inequalities in death — specific explanations of a general pattern?' *Lancet.* 5 May, pp.1003-6.

20. For further discussion of the issue of gender and CHD see, for example, Waldron, I. (1978), 'Type A behaviour pattern and CHD in men and women', *Social Science and Medicine,* Vol.12B, pp.167-70; Johnson, A. (1977), 'Sex differentiation in CHD — the explanatory role of primary risk factors', *Journal of Health and Social Behaviour,* Vol.18, pp.46-53; Price, L. (1983), 'Epidemiology, medical sociology and CHD', *Radical Community Medicine.* No.15; Bartley, M., Farrant, W., and Russell, J. (1986), *Women's Health and Heart Disease.* Women's Health Information Centre, London.

For a review of the evidence relating to CHD and Asians in Britain, see McKeigue, P.M., et. al. (1985), 'Diet and risk factors for coronary heart disease in Asians in North West London', *Lancet*, 16 November, pp.1086-9; Coronary Prevention Group (1986), *Coronary Heart Disease and Asians in Britain*. CPG, London.

21. St George (1983), op.cit. n.13 above.

22. Eyer, J. (1975), 'Hypertension as a disease of modern society', *International Journal of Health Services,* Vol.5, No.4, pp.539-58; Najman, J.M. (1980), 'Theories of disease causation and the concept of a general susceptibility. A review', *Social Science and Medicine,* Vol.14A, pp.231-7; St George (1983), op.cit. n.13 above; Markowe, H.L.J. et. al. (1985), 'Fibrinogen: a possible link between social class and CHD', *British Medical Journal,* Vol.291, pp.1312-14; Siegrist, J., Siegrist, K. and Weber, I. (1986), 'Sociological concepts in the etiology of chronic disease: the case of ischaemic heart disease', *Social Science and Medicine,* Vol.22, No.2, pp.247-53.

23. St George (1983), op.cit. n.22 above; Eyer (1975), op.cit. n.22 above.

24. Cook, D.G., Bartley, M.J., Cummins, R.O., and Shaper, A.G., (1982), 'Health of unemployed middle-aged men in Great Britain', *Lancet*. 5 June, Vol.1, pp.1290-4; Moser, K.A., Fox, A.J., Goldblatt, P.O. (1986), 'Stress and CHD: evidence of associations between unemployment and heart disease from the OPCS longitudinal study' in *Does Stress Cause Heart Attacks?*, Proceedings of a conference 18/19 November 1985. Coronary Prevention Group, London.

25. Brenner, M.M. (1971), 'Economic changes and heart disease mortality', *American Journal of Public Health,* Vol.61, p.606; Eyer, J. (1977), 'Prosperity as a cause of death', *International Journal of Health Services,* Vol.7, No.1, pp.125-51.

26. Theorell, T. (1986), 'Research on stress at work and risk of myocardial infarction', in *In Does Stress Cause Heart Attacks?* (1986), op.cit. n.24 above.; Karasek, R.A., Scott Russell, R., Theorell, T. (1982), 'Physiology of stress and regeneration in job related cardiovascular illness', *Journal of Human Stress,* Vol.8, No.29.

27. Friedman, M. and Rosenman, R. (1974), *Type A Behaviour and Your Heart*. Knopf, New York.

28. WHO Expert Committee (1982), op.cit. n.7 above.

29. Rose, G. (1981), 'Strategy of prevention: lessons from cardiovascular disease', *British Medical Journal,* Vol.282, pp.1847-51; Rose, G. (1985), 'Sick individuals and sick populations', *International Journal of Epidemiology,* Vol.14, No.1, pp.32-8.

30. Tunstall-Pedoe, H. (1984), 'Paunches and the prediction of CHD', *British Medical Journal,* Vol.288, No.6431, pp.1629-30.

31. Rose (1981), op.cit. n.29 above; WHO Expert Committee (1982), op.cit. n.7 above.

32. Rose (1981), ibid. n.29 above.

33. WHO Expert Committee (1986), op.cit. n.7 above.

34. For further discussion of this issue see Cannon, G. and Walker, C. (1986), *The Food Scandal.* Century, London. The NACNE report was subsequently published by the HEC: NACNE (1983), *Proposals for Nutrition Guidelines for Health Education in Britain.* HEC, London.

35. *Lancet* (1983), op.cit. n.6 above.

36. WHO Expert Committee (1986), op.cit. n.7 above.

37. Rose (1985), op.cit. n.29 above.

38. Jenkins, D. (1976), 'Recent evidence supporting psychological and social risk factors for coronary disease' (parts 1 and 2), *New England Journal of Medicine,* Vol.294, pp.987-94 and pp.1033-8.

39. Selye, H. (1956), *The Stress of Life.* McGraw-Hill, New York.

40. Marmot (1986), op.cit. Ch.1, n.4, above.

41. Ibid.

42. St George (1983), op.cit. n.13 above.

43. Eyer (1977), op.cit. n.25 above.

44. Manicom, C. (1981), 'Why doctors should face challenge of stress', *Health Education News,* November/December.

45. Health Education Council (1984), op.cit. n.7 above; Harding, J. and Price, L. (1986), *Preventing Coronary Heart Disease: a report of policies and initiatives in the UK.* Commissioned by and presented to the National Co-ordinating Committee on Coronary Heart Disease (NCCCHDP).

46. For further discussion of this issue see Farrant, W. (1986), *'Health for All' in the Inner City.* Paddington and North Kensington Health Education Unit, London.

47. WHO Expert Committee (1982), op.cit. n.7 above.

48. WHO Expert Committee (1986), op.cit. n.7 above.

Chapter 3

1. Farrant and Russell (1985), op.cit. Preface above.

2. Now renamed Public Affairs.

3. Now renamed Health Sciences.

4. 'Action makes the heart grow stronger' Radio 4 Series, 1983.

5. 'Plague of hearts' BBC2 Series, 1983.

6. Health Education Council (1982), *Annual Report 1981-1982,* HEC.

7. Health Education Council (1982), *Major Programmes for 1982-3,* HEC.

8. Health Education Council (1983), *Programmes for 1983-4,* HEC.

9. Farrant and Russell (1985), op.cit. Preface above.

10. St George, D. (1981), 'Who pulls the strings at the HEC?' *World Medicine,* 28 November, pp.51-3; Jones, W.T. and Grahame, H. (1973), *Health Education in Britain,* TUC Centenary, Institute of Occupational Health, London School of Hygiene and Tropical Medicine; Budd, J., Gray, P. and McCron, R. (1983), *The Tyne Tees Alcohol Education Campaign: an evaluation* HEC; Sutherland, I. (1987 forthcoming), *Health Education: half a policy 1968-86,* National Extension College, Cambridge.

11. Department of Health and Social Security (DHSS) (1981), *Avoiding Heart Attacks,* HMSO, London.

12. It was apparent that an overriding issue in the production of *Beating Heart Disease* was that of time: having to produce a booklet in time for the start of the TV series which it was supporting in print. The general constraints that time place on writing, consultation, design and research work need, therefore, constantly to be borne in mind. Our research on other HEC publications showed that such time constraints were not atypical.

13. If the Programme had been finalized, some of the evaluation of medical and scientific opinion would already have been translated into an HEC policy line and the job of the Publications Division and Medical Division would have been made that much easier. We discuss in Chapter 4 some of the problems resulting from the booklet's being written in advance of an HEC policy on, for example, quantified dietary goals.

14. Farrant and Russell (1985), op.cit. Preface above.

15. It is interesting to note that this structure (the HEOs Publication Panel), always recognized by the HEC and HEOs as somewhat tokenistic in its composition and ability to influence decision making, has since been disbanded. Although new structures have now been set up for HEC/HEO consultation, the failure of the HEC to take account of HEOs views on publications is still a major dissatisfaction expressed by HEOs.

16. Leathar, D.S. (1981), *The Use of Mass Media Health Education Campaigns in Scotland,* Appendix 2 to summary of report of the HEC Working Group on evaluation of health education.

17. A former HEC research officer (in a personal communication) has suggested a similar interpretation of the use the HEC makes of pretesting research: 'it . . . became a confidence booster, legitimiser or justifier, usually when it was too late to change anything'.

Chapter 4

1. Rakusen, J. (1982), 'Feminism and the politics of health', *Medicine in Society,* Vol.8, No.1, pp.17-25.

2. Health Education Council (1983), op.cit. Ch.3, n.8, above.

3. WHO Expert Committee (1982), *Prevention of Coronary Heart Disease,* Technical Report Series No.678. World Health Organisation, Geneva.

4. BBC (1983), 'Insight into health', *Insight Information.*

5. See the HEC/SHEG leaflet 'The flurodiation of public water supplies'.

6. In the final report of the Health Education Publications Project (Farrant and Russell 1985 op.cit. Preface above) we cite some isolated instances in which HEC publications *have* taken a stand against current social policy. One such example (produced subsequent to the publication of *Beating Heart Disease*) was the inclusion in the booklet *Food for Thought* (1984) of a full-page spread entitled 'Food and profit: healthier eating for all requires changes in the food industry'. This was accompanied by another full-page spread on food labelling, which encouraged readers to lobby food manufacturers, Members of Parliament, and the Minister of Agriculture to bring about improved standards of food labelling. We noted that the less-individualistic orientation of *Food for Thought,* in comparison with the normal range of HEC publications, could be attributed to a number of factors, including the background and perspective of the author (a social scientist); the fact that the booklet (which was produced to accompany a Channel 4 TV series of the same title) was never intended to become a long-term addition to the HEC publications

list; and the involvement of an HEC officer who had the time, commitment and nutritional expertise to defend up to ministerial level, in the face of considerable opposition from the food industry, the scientific and ethical rationale for addressing the issue of food and profit.

As we predicted in our final report, this wider perspective was not retained in the DHSS-commissioned booklet *Eating for a Healthier Heart* (1985) which superseded *Food for Thought*. *Eating for a Healthier Heart* was produced by the HEC on conjunction with the British Nutrition Foundation (a body which represents the interests of the food industry) to publicize the recommendations of the 1984 Report of the Committee on Medical Aspects of Food Policy, Diet and Cardiovascular Disease. Considerable media publicity was given to the intervention by the Government and the food industry in the drafting of *Eating for a Healthier Heart*.

Advocacy of collective action reappears, however, in the more recent HEC booklet on general nutrition, *Healthy Eating*. A full-page spread which has the title 'Action' provides suggestions for collective action aimed at putting pressure on workplaces, schools, NHS premises and food retailers to produce more healthy food, and lobbying for more information on food labels.

Analysis of the production of these more recent publications is beyond the scope of this paper. We mention them here merely to illustrate the shifting boundaries of the constraints under which the HEC is working, and the element of flexibility in interpreting these constraints.

7. Farrant and Russell (1985), op.cit. Preface above.

8. See, for example, the reports of surveys by Ann Cartwright and her colleagues at the Institute for Social Studies in Medical Care that challenge the assumption that people from social classes IV and V do not want information about their health (e.g. Cartwright, A., 1979, *The Dignity of Labour,* Tavistock, London).

9. Wilding, P. (1982), *Professional Power and Social Welfare.* Routledge & Kegan Paul, London.

10. The standard arguments for the use of readability tests, and the confused logic behind such arguments, are clearly expressed in a paper prepared by an HEO on 'a simplified Reading East Estimation method for health educators' which states:

> Many leaflets and other materials produed for the general public can only be understood by a minority. This paradox has been shown by applying standard readability scores, so evidently much material is not being tested for readability before being distributed. This costly and nonsensical problem demands a solution.

This suggests that a readability score alone will determine whether or not material can be understood by the general public. In fact, the most commonly used readability measure in health education (the Flesch score) simply measures the number of syllables per 100 words and the average number of words per sentence. The test fails to take account of a variety of other factors that will, of course, influence readability; legibility of print; use of illustrations and colour; conceptual difficulty of text; organization of material; motivation of the reader; and age, circumstance and experience of the reader, for example (for further discussion of these issues see Harrison, C. (1980), *Readability in Classrooms,* Cambridge University Press).

11. Sutherland, I. (1979), 'History and background', in I. Sutherland, (ed.), *Health education; perspectives and choices.* George Allen and Unwin, London.

12. *British Medical Journal,* (1982), 'New thoughts for the Health Education Council' (editorial), *British Medical Journal,* Vol.285, No.6357, pp.1761-2.

13. WHO Expert Committee (1982), op.cit. Ch.2, n.7, above.

14. Health Education Council (1983), op.cit. Ch.3, n.8 above.

15. *Health Education News* (1981), 'Heart disease risks ignored'. HEC, September/October.

16. Office of Health Economics (1982), *Coronary Heart Disease — the scope for prevention,* No.73 in a series of papers on current health problems.

17. Manicom (1981), op.cit. Ch.2, n.4, above.

Chapter 5

1. Graham, H. (1976), 'Smoking in preganancy: the attitudes of expectant mothers', *Social Science and Medicine,* Vol.10, pp.399-405.

2. Richards, N.D. (1975), 'Methods and effectiveness of health education: the past, present and future of social scientific involvement', *Social Science and Medicine,* Vol.9, pp.141-56.

3. Health Education Studies Unit (1982), *Final Report on the Patient Project* (September 1977 to November 1982). HEC, London.

4. e.g.: Tuckett, D., Boulton, M., Olson, C. and Williams, A. (1985), *Meetings Between Experts, an approach to sharing ideas in medical consultations.* Tavistock, London; Graham, H. (1985), *Caring for the Family; a short report of the study of the organization of health resources and responsibilities in 102 families with pre-school children.* HEC, London; Cornwall, J. (1984), *Hard Earned Lives: accounts of health and illness from East London.*

Tavistock, London; Charles, N. and Kerr, M. (1984), *Attitudes Towards the Feeding and Nutrition of Young Children: report to the HEC,* HEC; Graham (1976), op.cit. n.1 above; Graham, H. and McKee, L. (1980), *The First Months of Motherhood,* No.3 in a Monograph Series, HEC, London; CUE (1977), *Positive Health: report on 16 group discussions,* prepared for HEC by the British Market Research Bureau Ltd, London; Dorn, N. (1980), 'Alcohol in teenage cultures: a materialist approach to youth cultures, drinking and health education', *Health Education Journal,* Vol.39, No.3, pp.67-73; Pill, R. and Stott, N.C.M. (1982), 'Concepts of illness causation and responsibility: some preliminary data from a sample of working class mothers', *Social Science and Medicine,* Vol.16, pp.43-52.

5. e.g. Hubley, J. (1979), *A Community Development Approach to Health Education in a Multiply-deprived Community in Scotland,* paper presented at 10th International Conference on Health Education, London; Rosenthal, H. (1980), *Health and Community Work: some new approaches,* paper commissioned by the King Edward's Hospital Fund for London; London Community Health Resource (1983), *Community Initiatives in Health Education,* LVSC, London; Watt, A. (1984), *Community Development and Health Education,* Community Health Initiatives Resource Unit; Somerville, G. (1984), *Community Development in Health: addressing the confusions,* report of a conference organised by the King's Fund in collaboration with the London Community Health Resource and the Community Health Initiatives Resource Unit, London Community Health Resource, LVSC, London; Drennan, V. (1986), *Effective Health Education in the Inner City,* report of a feasibility study examining community development approaches for health education officers and health education departments, Paddington and North Kensington Health Authority.

6. Farrant, W. and Russell, J. (1983), *Beating Heart Disease: a case study in the production of Health Education Council publications,* HEC, London.

7. Graham (1976), op.cit. n.1 above.

8. Graham (1985), op.cit. n.4 above.

9. Hall, J. (1976), *Subjective Measures of Quality of Life in Britain: 1971-1975,* Polytechnic of North London, (formerly of the Survey Unit, SSRC); CUE (1977), op.cit. n.4 above; Pill, R. and Stott, N. (1980), *Health Beliefs in an Urban Community,* Department of General Practice, Welsh National School of Medicine.

10. e.g.: Betts, G. (1984), *Health in Glyndon: report of a survey on health,* Greenwich Community Health Council, London; Catford Community Health

Project (1985), *Evaluation Report* Catford Community Health Project, London; Lambeth Health Bus (1984), *Lambeth Health Bus: a report,* Lambeth Community Health Services, London; Tower Hamlets Health Education Unit (1984), *The Spitalfields Health Survey,* Tower Hamlets Health Authority.

11. e.g. Graham, (1985), op.cit. n.4 above; Cole-Hamilton, I. and Lang, T. (1986), *Tightening Belts: a report on the impact of poverty on food,* London Food Commission.

12. Murcott, A. (1983), ' "Its a pleasure to cook for him"': food, meal times and gender in some South Wales households' in: E. Garmarnikow et. al. (eds.) *The Public and the Private,* Heinemann, London; Charles and Kerr (1984), op.cit. n.4 above; Women and Food Group (1982), *Women's Health and Food,* Women's Health Information Centre, London.

13. We would hypothesize that many research findings on levels of information in health education materials are methodologically flawed in their failure to distinguish between people talking for themselves and for other people. For example, one business executive whom we interviewed said:

    My worry is that the average guy would get half way through and not get to the end, and he'll be confused by it — with no clear idea of how it applies to him . . . you may have to forgo the arguments and just say saturated fat is bad for you.

    Even though, for himself, this respondent said he would want both sides of the argument. Rakusen, in research for the Health Education Publications Project on women's information needs on the menopause, noted how women unanimously wanted a lot of information for themselves, but some assumed that *other* women would only be prepared to read a short leaflet.

14. Farrant, W. and Russell, J. (1984),*Information about the Menopause: lay and professional reactions to a draft publication,* Health Education Publications Project, University of London Institute of Education.

15. Dickinson, R. (1983), *The Health Education Council's Guide to a Healthy Pregnancy: a survey of users,* Centre for Mass Communication Research, Leicester; Dickinson, R. and Rocheron, Y. (1985),*Publicising Pregnancy Care: an evaluation of the pregnancy book campaign,* Centre for Mass Communication Research, Leicester.

16. *Lancet* (1983), op.cit. Ch.2, n.6, above.

17. McCron (1982), *Differences between Commercial Sales Campaigns and Health Education Campaigns,* Appendix 1 to Summary Report of the HEC Working Group on Evaluation of Health Education.

18. This possibility of turning people off future health education messages again highlights the fundamental difference between health education and the commercial selling of a message. As Eiser has explained (HEC seminar 1981), in marketing terms, if an advertising campaign attracts 1 million people and turns off 11 million, it is still seen in evaluation terms as a success. In other words, as long as a commercial campaign achieves a net positive result, it is of little consequence if it alienates as many or more potential customers as it attracts. This cannot apply to health education.

Chapter 6

1. DHSS (1981), op.cit. Ch.3, n.11, above. At the time of publication of this paper, DHSS are about to launch a major national CHD prevention campaign.

2. See Harding and Price (1986), op.cit. Ch.2, n.45 above and Health Education Council (1984), op.cit. Ch.2, n.7 above.

3. Price, L. (1983), 'Epidemiology, medical sociology and CHD', *Radical Community Medicine,* Autumn pp.10-15.

4. Farrant and Russell (1985), op.cit. Preface above; Farrant, W. and Russell, J. (1986), 'Community initiatives in health education publications: a role for health education of officers?' in S. Rodmell and A. Watt, (1986), *The Politics of Health Education*. Routledge & Kegan Paul, London.

5. Farrant and Russell (1985), op.cit. Preface above.

6. World Health Organization Regional Office for Europe (1985), *Targets for Health for All 2000.* WHO, Copenhagen.